# Healing Massage for Babies and Toddlers

Y

To the mother in all of us

# Healing Massage for Babies and Toddlers

Julia Woodfield

Floris Books

Translated from German by Anna Cardwell

First published as *Gesunde Kinder fördern
kranke Kinder heilen* by Novalis Verlag AG Schaffhausen in 1996
First published in English in 2004 by Floris Books
© 2004 Julia Woodfield, 1996
Translation © 2004 Floris Books

Julia Woodfield has asserted her right under the
Copyright, Designs and Patents Act 1988
to be identified as the Author of this Work.

British Library CIP Data available

ISBN 0–86315–456–5

Printed in Great Britain
by Cromwell Press, Trowbridge

# Contents

# Foreword

Our attitude towards newborn babies and the way we treat and care for them has changed radically in recent years. During the '50s hygiene was given the foremost consideration; we now know, however, that bodily contact and emotional attention are of prime importance for the newborn. Even the best nursing or medical care cannot be a substitute for tender touch and the feeling of security and acceptance.

Modern medical technology is now able to save newborn babies who only a few years ago, would not have survived. But it cannot fulfil the psychological needs of a sick child. Increasingly, doctors and nurses are aware of this, and some medical practices are being questioned. Efforts are being made towards changing the focal point from overly material and technical practices to a more holistic approach; towards the improved observation of the psychological and spiritual needs of the patient.

Today we know more than ever about the psychological needs of a baby. Birth and the experiences of the first months have lasting effects. Although there are already some trends towards acknowledging the psychological needs of a baby, a lot more can be done. There is a big discrepancy between what has been recognized and published and what is, in fact, practised. In this book I am going to deal with complimentary therapies for premature and sick babies and toddlers, focusing on tactile stimulation (i.e. touching).

This book describes a few easy and effective methods that can be used in hospitals or at home, in conjunction with conventional medicines. These can be used by parents, staff and other carers. I hope I can inspire and encourage people who want to care for, and heal, sick children.

Staying in hospital is a big psychological strain for babies and can severely disrupt the mother-child relationship. Intensive care often has traumatic consequences. We know from adult psychotherapy that early childhood experiences can have lasting effects on the life of a person.

Sensitive nurses in Western countries are not happy with the over-emphasis on painful, invasive measures for their patients. In 1992 in Poland this theme was dealt with at the "World Conference for Prenatal and Perinatal Psychology."

It is a theme which comes up in practically all the courses I give to paediatric nurses, midwives and maternal counsellors, and is invariably a source of great concern. I know there are a large number of carers who long for the chance to bring some humanity and warmth into high-tech medicine.

# Foreword for parents

When I started writing about tactile stimulation for babies I was thinking more of a collection of notes and documents for paediatric nurses, midwives and health visitors. But I soon realized that parents remain the most important people for the newborn — even when the newborn needs intensive hospital care. So I increasingly aimed my work at parents. Only when a child receives both professional care and attachment to their mother will they become healthy. The child needs the co-operation of medical experts and parents.

There is no doubt that nowadays babies can be saved who would not have survived one or two decades ago. But new, highly specialized, technical medicine contains a risk of one-sidedness. Despite obvious success it remains clear to many parents and specialists that biological survival alone is not enough. Science and technology can damage if we forget fundamental psychological needs. Sick children need their mother's love, attention and touch as well as life-saving medical help. For healthy children most maternity wards offer 'rooming in.' However, a premature or sick child not only has to cope with the stressful and painful experience of medical intervention, but also with separation from its mother — the worst thing that can happen to a newborn child.

In the children's wards and intensive care units of many hospitals much has changed in the last few years. Parents are now allowed access to intensive care units because it is accepted that babies need their mothers, and that they prosper and recover better when their fundamental need for loving bodily contact and tender touch is fulfilled. Thus many doctors and nurses strive towards integrating parents into the healing process.

Parents are not condemned to watch helplessly and passively. If your child needs intensive care there is now the possibility to support and accompany it in its difficult journey. You can give it what it needs beside the life-saving medical measures — your vital loving attention, touch and kindness.

Trust your instinctive feelings for your child. Follow your urge to be near your baby. Talk to the responsible doctor and nurse; nurses usually understand how difficult the separation is for you.

Discuss your intention to be with your child as much as possible and to give your child lots of bodily contact. Clarify with the doctor what is possible from a medical point of view. You may be shown the "kangaroo method" or gentle massage. In Part III of this book you can learn a few different, easy tactile treatments that are suitable for your child even if it has to remain in intensive care.

If you want to help your sick child right now, turn directly to Part V (page 87), practical methods. The information contained in Part I about development and physical processes is not necessary for what your child needs at this point. Intellectual knowledge will not determine the quality of treatment, but rather the intensity of care. Touch is probably the oldest way of helping a suffering, frightened person. You do not need to have studied physiotherapy or have a degree in massage to give comfort, encouragement and love with your hands.

# Preface

It is not enough to treat the physical pain.
The whole person suffers, and the
whole person has to be treated.[1]

New medical findings do not always mean progress. It is often possible to do more than is good for us, and we are confronted with the question of limits. The possibilities of medical technology put the people concerned in the difficult position of having to decide about life and death, about questionable therapies or about treatments with serious side effects. Many are shocked by the influence and role of medical technology, not because it is bad by itself, but because it neglects other fundamental factors. The fascination and belief in science make us too one-sided. Treatment in surgeries and hospitals is almost exclusively concerned with the body and our attention is turned towards symptoms that can be seen and measured. The diagnosis appears to be more important, and takes up more time, than the treatment. Patients encourage this tendency. They want immediate removal of their ailment, without any personal participation and without having to change their lifestyle.

Many specialists and laymen are troubled by this imbalance. We need to consider the psychological needs, as well as the bodily needs, of sick people — both children and adults. Fear, worry and loneliness hinder the process of healing. We can only really help the patient by accompanying them in the less obvious areas of thought and feeling. They need our emotional attention as a fellow human being.

There are, and always have been doctors who realize this. A good example is Dr Cicely Saunders, the founder of the hospice movement. In her hospital she works according to these basic principles and has inspired thousands. Her theory of 'total pain' aims towards helping patients on all levels. The whole team strives towards the highest possible amount of life quality and dignity for the patient. Relatives help and form part of the team.

Saunder describes 'total pain' as:

| | |
|---|---|
| *body pain* | illness |
| *emotional pain* | feelings of helplessness, isolation, fear |
| *social pain* | fear and worry about family, finances, living etc. |
| *spiritual pain* | longing for security finding meaning to life |

Ideally, holistic healing touches all these areas. Age does not matter in these fundamental matters. Newborns feel and react in the same ways as adults or terminally-ill people — they suffer from one-sided therapy lacking emotional attention, warmth and empathy. We are an inseparable whole. Everything is connected and intertwined in a complex way. If something is happening in even a small part of the body, it affects the whole body and is connected with feelings. On the other hand every feeling is mirrored in the body. This knowledge sounds banal, but we seem to have forgotten it.

While striving to help it is good to observe which level we are dealing with — the purely physical, or with another subjective, psychological-spiritual level, inaccessible through logic. The 'deeper' we go the better. A phenomenon of healing is that the invisible levels of feeling and thinking are stronger than the bodily processes. We cannot speak of healing when we just remove the symptoms, thus leaving the patient alone with their psychological needs, and ignoring their feelings and fears, however irrational they may seem.

> *Holistic healing recognizes and takes into account the dominating influence of the emotions and feelings on bodily processes.*

This attitude is useful in all areas of medicine from birth onwards. Not only Saunders, but many doctors think like this and show that this attitude is possible to implement. The following chapters have evolved from this point of view.

# I. Birth and Fundamental Needs

## Birth

Breath is stronger than a sword — just as the mind is stronger than the flesh.[2]

It is almost impossible to think about a newborn's situation without discussing its birth. Actually we should start even earlier with the pregnancy and the time before conception as they influence the later life. So where does it start? Is it not a cycle without end — a passing on through generations? It is clear that we are responsible for our descendants long before they appear — we carry this responsibility both individually and collectively. The food we eat, our state of mind and our lifestyle are factors that play a part in new life. There were some cultures which took special notice of this fact. Pregnant women were specially cared for and revered, and surrounded by beautiful things. Music was played for them (and thus for the unborn baby), myths and heroic tales were read to them. Ugly and frightening impressions were kept away from them if possible. In our culture there are more and more women who barely look after themselves and expect to produce a child while studying, having a career and doing daily tasks. There are also few couples who consciously prepare for conception. We teach adolescents all sorts of things, but do not prepare them for the most important task of becoming a parent. This should be a necessity, as we now live isolated in small families and no longer have extended families whose example we can follow.

How a mother and child experience the birth and the first hours after is very important. This experience plays a part in their relationship and the later development of the child. Right after birth the important process of bonding starts.

### The first hours in the child's life

Normally a newborn is wide awake during the first hour after the birth. "Wide alert state" is the medical term for this condition.

If a newborn is held and surrounded with a peaceful atmosphere it usually calms down very quickly and relaxes. It is amazing to watch how its facial expression changes from the effort of the birth to a smooth pink colour. Its eyes are open and inquisitive. It is wonderful to look into a child's deeply questioning and knowing eyes. The child appears not to miss anything. It can maintain eye contact and evidently listens to the voice talking to it. It has differentiated reactions to the way it is treated: sighing and sucking when it feels good, or reacting angrily if treated roughly or without feeling. The idea that newborns cannot see, feel or smell properly has long been superseded by new evidence.

As long as the mother has not been sedated during birth the child will not be affected and will start to make its first contact with the outside world shortly after it has been born, by looking for its mother's breast.

Painkillers are a theme worthy of consideration. The way we treat pain during the last phase of birth sets the scene for the future. Painkillers not only influence the physical processes of the person giving birth, but also the behaviour of the mother and child after the birth.

> If you want to use the biological readiness of mother and child, you must bear in mind that analgesics and narcotics can affect the state of awareness of newborns. Thus Kron (9, 1996) and Newton & Newton (1962) showed that even four days after birth babies of medicated mothers sucked significantly slower and with less pressure than their non-medicated controls. The frequently quoted suckling problems of babies can in a number of cases be partly traced to medication, or to a delayed start in breast-feeding.[3]

Babies of sedated mothers are also often suckled later because they are not awake enough after the birth to look for the mother's breast.

I know from my experience and from births I have assisted that painkillers are often given as part of the procedure, without the women asking for them. We know from many women that giving birth without painkillers is not only possible, but also natural. Provided that we support and accompany the mother emotionally, labour can be mastered without painkillers. In fact, many women describe a euphoric state while giving birth. They experience a conscious state of exceptional energy and joy despite heavy labour.

This heightened state of awareness and the feeling of happiness are due to body chemistry. There is a pain-regulating system in the organism of all humans and vertebrate animals. The body deals with pain by increasing the production of endorphins. These are endogenous morphines which block the transmission of pain in the spine and can induce euphoric feelings — a fact that, if known by women in advance, could well reduce their fears about giving birth. Many women opt for a caesarean birth because they are frightened of labour pains, not realizing that the post-operative discomfort and pain caused by a caesarean section may be worse.

The body is naturally capable of managing the birthing process. This is also reported by experienced midwives like Ina May Gaskin and specialists like Michael Odent.[4] For many years they have pointed out that birthing women instinctively do the right thing and can allow the internal intelligence of their body to take over, if they are emotionally supported and surrounded by an atmosphere of intimacy and trust. Women supported in this way automatically take up a position that is anatomically correct and physiologically helpful, if their feeling for their body and their psychological state is not damaged.

An atmosphere of security is necessary to maintain unblocked "biological intelligence." Keeping the right balance requires sensitivity. Women can react with interrupted labour and other problems when they have a midwife they do not like, or alternatively with quick cervix dilation when the shift changes or a trusted doctor appears.

John Kennel conducted an extensive controlled study at the Davis hospital, Houston, Texas into the influence of continual emotional care during birth. The results show without doubt what a big influence the care of a female birthing partner — a *doula* — can be for the woman giving birth (doula comes from Greek and means an experienced women supporting and educating a young mother):

> The study showed that the continuous presence of an experienced female assistant reduced the necessity for caesarean-sections markedly. Moreover, the births were shorter, less interventions were needed and there were fewer perinatal problems for the foetus and the newborn.[6]

The mother's preparation for birth as well as her inner attitude towards it also influence her subjective feeling of pain and the birthing process. The greatest obstacle is unconscious and raw fear. It can literally block the birth and be the reason behind contractions stopping, an undilating cervix or spasmodic contractions. The body mirrors unconscious psychological problems and thus cannot fulfil its task. People working with birthing mothers can experience many examples of this kind.

There is one couple I have never forgotten: in an antenatal course we did an exercise in which couples had to observe the feelings that emerged when they thought about the impending birth. One of the couples had a strong feeling of uneasiness. They both worked in the clinic and with the people they had chosen for the birth. He was a paediatrician, she was a nurse. The pregnant woman noticed that she was worried she would embarrass herself in front of her colleagues by screaming or other 'difficult' behaviour. The couple realized that the conditions were not ideal, but felt that they 'owed' their workmates the birth as proof of their trust in them. One week before the due date the woman's cervix was soft and 2 cm dilated. The doctor thought the birth would be quick and easy. At the start of the birth at home the woman still had good contractions, but as soon as she reached the hospital she had difficulties: her contractions kept stopping, and her cervix stopped dilating. After many difficult hours they decided a caesarean was the only option.

The physical conditions for an easy birth had all been there. But the woman had not taken her concerns seriously, and her repressed fears led to problems. It is a true phenomenon that psychological forces are stronger than physiological processes. It is always good to listen to the quiet inner voice warning us. This voice comes from deep inner knowledge and cannot be taken seriously enough.

If fathers ask me what they can do for their wives during the birth when they feel helpless, I always believe that they know their wife best and know how to encourage and calm her. Whatever encourages and calms is the best for her. For most women the presence of their partner is encouraging.

## Practical tips for a natural birth

### Some good remedies

It is good if the mother and birth partner have a range of ideas and remedies to use for specific situations. Not every remedy works for every woman, and often one remedy will only work temporarily during a specific birthing phase.

### The following can help withstand painkillers

Firstly, the ability to understand and allow the women giving birth to have pain, strong emotions and feelings like fear, anger, hopelessness;

Secondly, the use of natural remedies that help to soothe. There are many natural remedies instead of painkillers to ease the opening phase.

## The wonderful effect of water

### Poultice for the perineum

.Hot, damp poultice (large sanitary towel) is placed onto the perineum

Immerse a large sanitary towel in boiling water or camomile tea, as hot as the woman can bear but still finds comfortable, place it on the perineum and cover with a dry cloth.

The husband or companion can press it down with their hand. Women find these compresses very soothing.

The following are helpful:
— Warmth, to help relaxation;
— Camomile, to loosen cramps and soothe pain;
— Touch and human attentiveness.

### Washing

Rub the back and stomach with a cloth. It is possible to add camomile or a dash of vinegar to aid relaxation.

### Bathing

The woman in labour has a warm bath.

Water can be magical. Most women feel better in the warmth and weightlessness of water. You can add a few drops of essential oils, such as lavender, clary sage, rose or jasmine. All these plants are suitable for birth — they relax the body, and revive or support the contractions. It is important to observe the reactions of the woman. Do not leave her alone in the bathtub. The woman giving birth should get up and then get back into the water regularly. The change between warmth and cold rouses the body and gives the impulse for better contractions. I was once told by a women who knew a lot about Africa that in some areas of Ghana the mothers giving birth are washed alternately with hot and ice-cold water.

### Steam baths
#### Steam bath with herbs

A steam bath can be very soothing for the pelvis and prepares the perineum for extreme stretching. It is very simple to do. Take a normal plastic bowl and fill it three-quarters full with boiling water. Add two to three tablespoons of camomile, weak Melissa or rue (*Ruta graveolens*) tea. Balance the plastic bowl in the toilet so the woman can sit comfortably above it. It is important that the legs and upper body of the woman giving birth are kept warm. It is advisable to wear long, thick socks. Warmth is important for birthing, cold induces cramp, and any kind of cramp, whether physical or psychological, is counterproductive.

## *The effect of touch*

### *Massage*

> Massage helps to relax and supports all physiological processes such as breathing, circulation and so on.

Massage has proven itself to be helpful during birth. It can be practised by the midwife, husband or birthing partner. The needs of the woman should be taken into account: feet, back and lower back, perineum and thigh (particularly the inner side) are comforting to have massaged. The erogenous zones of the inner thigh work reflectively onto the sexual organs. Massaging the perineum with oil containing vitamin E during pregnancy improves elasticity of the perineum muscles. For an effective massage have a look at the tips given in the chapter about baby massage. Couples who think massage would be a good way of supporting natural birth should spend some time practising it together beforehand. The father can effectively help his wife in the often long opening phase. But not everyone feels comfortable with massage; in our western culture it is still strange for many people.

### *Holding, resting hands*

Most husbands and birthing partners naturally touch and hold the woman giving birth. Laying a hand on the body is probably the oldest form of healing and a natural expression of sympathy. Most women experience holding and laying hands on painful parts during contractions, like the lower back or the pubic bone, as a great comfort. We impart energy and new courage through our hands. The intensity and depth of this can change depending on the concentration and sensitivity with which we observe the processes happening to the woman. The woman will notice any distractedness, for example if we are fascinated by the foetal monitoring unit and do not notice the human level.

### *Movement, position*

Circling the hips during contractions:

> *Moving the hips during contractions.*

The midwife or husband should encourage the woman giving birth to move her hips. At the same time one hand is placed on her lower back, the other gently on her stomach above the pubic bone. When a contraction starts, slowly rotate the pelvis and ask the woman to keep her knees relaxed, so that she is not standing on tense legs. If the woman is kneeling on all fours, do the same: place one hand on her lower back, the other on her stomach, and move her pelvis. It helps, even if the women do not want to believe it!

Many hospitals have a medicine ball for the woman to sit and rotate her pelvis. This has the same effect and works best if there is something to hold on to, for example a rope, rings or a bar.

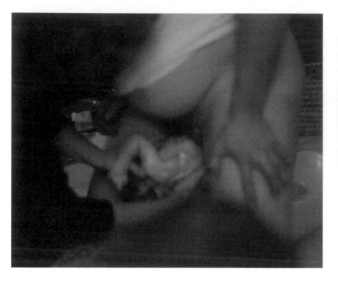

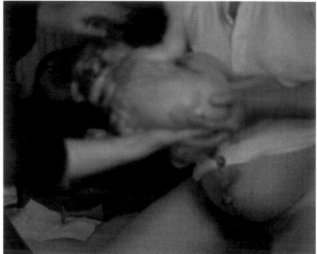

*Positions*

Positions should be changed again and again! Some women will instinctively choose a physiologically correct position. But others need encouragement and impetus. She might not believe that she can move, but if she manages after some support and help she will usually be very grateful and feel some relief.

We know that lying on your back is not a good position. Despite its physiological inappropriateness woman are often told to lie in bed during the opening phase. Liselotte Kuntner has written an excellent book about the effect of position on birth.[6]

## The best support — breathing

Breathing is the best support for anyone giving birth, and most women learn the techniques in antenatal classes. But once the contractions get very heavy during the middle and end phases they often forget what they have learnt. It is important that the midwife or husband remind the woman to breathe out deeply, and even join in breathing. Breathing out should be stressed. The effect can be enhanced greatly through the right mental images. This means linking a thought or inner picture to the breathing, for example:

Imagine with every exhalation that your body is becoming heavy and relaxed.

Or: Your body is opening like the bud of a flower.

Or: Your breath is flowing into every cell of your lower body and making it penetrable and soft etc.

### Using voice

While giving antenatal classes I found that many women were worried they would start screaming and embarrass themselves. It is impossible to overestimate the obstructing effect of such fears. Women should be made to feel that it is all right to make a noise or scream. If she starts screeching hysterically or fearfully we can encourage her to say vowels like Aaaaahh or Ooooohh from the depths of her stomach. We can show her how and 'sing' with her until her fear subsides. Singing long vowels during contractions is a great help. It gives a feeling of primal energy and control and guarantees deep breathing.[7]

### Calcium as a painkiller

Adelle Davis, an expert in the areas of health and nutrition, recommends that her clients:

> ... take with a glass of whole milk enough tablets to supply 2000 milligrams of calcium between the time labour started and the time they arrived at the hospital. Many had easy deliveries and some declared that they had experienced almost no pain. Most were convinced that the extra calcium had been helpful.[8]

All of the remedies mentioned above are easy to apply and can be used by a partner or friend. Most husbands are happy to actively take part in the process, and it gives them deep satisfaction to support their wife practically as well as emotionally.

These remedies can be useful especially

with long births, enabling a birth without tranquillizers as crisis points are overcome. There are always some crises to get stuck in. Sometimes just a small thing can bring about a change, bringing encouragement or mobilizing secret energy stores. These are often the moments that decide between a 'natural' birth and a birth with intervention and technology.

### Music

Most people react to music. I always take some tapes and a small tape recorder with me to births in hospital. Music changes the whole

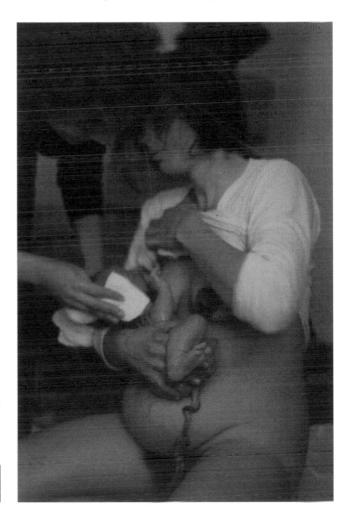

atmosphere in the room and often the husband benefits too. At a home birth one women asked for her favourite music to be played continually, because, as she said, she did not feel the pain anymore.

*Summary*

Everything that promotes a woman's trust, calms her, gives her energy and creates an atmosphere of protection should be offered. Only some of the possibilities have been described. Substituting heavy drugs and unnecessary technological interventions with patience and natural remedies has its rewards. It makes it possible for the woman giving birth to stay awake and aware for one of the most intense and happiest experiences in her life. The birth can become a high point in her life as well as an important developmental step towards the new task of becoming a mother. The sense of achievement improves her confidence and gives her security for breastfeeding and mothering.

And very importantly: the newborn is born more alert and has a better start in life. We as helpers can contribute a lot towards such a peaceful start.

# The infant's basic needs

## *The principle of continuity*

The circumstances in the womb are ideal for protecting the growing child:

— weightlessness and security (weightlessness relieves the organism)
— neither hunger nor thirst
— constant, ideal temperature
— movement and rocking
— constant touch through the walls of the uterus every time the mother or the foetus moves

The foetus moves almost continually in the womb. The skin, which senses before any other organ, is touched, stroked and stimulated every time the mother moves. The growing child knows neither hunger nor cold nor abandonment. After the birth these ideal circumstances change at once. The security of the womb is left and separation is complete. Interaction with the outer world and all its challenges begins. Suddenly there are loud, frightening noises, heat, cold, hunger, the danger of falling and the terrible feeling of abandonment.[9]

Being born means separation — a theme that occupies us as an adult and throughout life. The new, outer circumstances of the environment are a fact and a necessary challenge. The infant has to adapt and begin its independent life, but there are qualitatively different ways this can happen! What a difference if we can still give the child a sense of security and can accompany it during this experience.

We know that conditions found in the womb are still good for the child after birth. Jean Liedloff uses the term "Continuum Principle" and shows magnificently in her book how lonely babies are in our "highly civilized" culture because we do not carry them against our bodies anymore.[10]

Warmth, touch, rocking, being held, bodily contact and stroking are basic needs of the baby Daily care and breastfeeding alone are not enough. The newborn needs loving attententiveness and gentle touch from its carer.

> *It is helpful for the newborn if we can create similar conditions to those it experienced before birth*

## Bonding

The healthy development of a baby relies on its connection with a single trusted person. A reliable — or even better a deep loving relationship — is the basis for the healthy development of the individual, and gives basic trust and self-respect. On the other hand the lack of such a person leads to pain, loss of a feeling of self and problems in later life.

If a natural birth is not disturbed by complications from the mother or child or medical intervention, then the process of bonding begins straight after birth, which is another reason to consciously abstain from painkillers.

### Astonishment

Once the baby is born the mother needs a few moments to admire it with astonishment. As long as the baby is fine and there is no need for interference this moment should be allowed to happen. Often it is bypassed by the urge to act straight after the birth. We have lost the knack of waiting, letting things happen and trusting the mother to do the right thing.

If we leave the mother with the baby she will usually welcome it lovingly and with admiration using a high sing-song voice. Then she will touch and stroke it gently with her fingertips, before grasping it more firmly and drawing it towards her.

I know a woman who arranged with the midwife to let her do as she wished during the birth. She took a lot of time to welcome the child, to hold it and pick it up. It was an impressing and satisfying experience which she often talked about.

### Bonding behaviour

The child brings with it the ability to interact with the world. Through its behaviour it arouses a reaction from its carers, and looks for a bond with a regular person — usually the mother. This response is called *bonding behaviour*.

It is necessary for a newborn to have a relationship with its personal environment. A human being can only find out who he is by mirroring himself against someone who reacts to him. The newborn is well equipped to get this attention by awakening strong feelings of love and care in us.

Instinctively we respond to this bonding behaviour. We look at the child, smile, talk and make funny faces and noises to make it laugh. We stroke, rock and hold it. Normally this behaviour is instinctive and playful.

If the regular person does not respond to the child, for whatever reasons, in the long-term or temporarily, then the child will receive the basic feeling it is neither loved nor loveable.

## A regular person

The baby needs at least one or two regular people — usually both parents. In the daily rhythm of feeding, changing and playful interaction they fulfil the needs of the baby and deepen the relationship.

> Only by giving the baby our love can it develop its "I", the trust that it is not helpless and a positive feeling of itself.
>
> This feeling that the baby achieves by interacting with its personal environment leads to a certain type of relationship or bonding behaviour, as the experts say. It has been found that the bonding behaviour with the regular person lasts at least till age six (this is as far as it has been studied). That means the early, affective behaviour has long-lasting consequences for its later development.[11]

## The bonding process with hospitalized infants

The bonding process is made more difficult for sick or premature newborns who have to be observed or remain in intensive care. In this case it is often not the mother who feeds and cares for the baby, but a whole team of people that changes in shifts according to the time of day and week. Even in the space of one shift the baby will be looked after by different people. In a few hours many faces will look at it, touch and hold it. Many things that happen to it are painful. It is difficult for a child in such a situation to bond with anybody and develop trust.

This fact became clear to me when I worked for a week in an infant care unit, teaching new mothers and staff baby massage:

There was a five-week-old baby on that ward whose mother had been transferred to a bigger hospital directly after the birth. The baby was born on its due date and was healthy, but could not leave the hospital as nobody was at home to look after it.

The nurses loved and spoiled the baby because it had been there longer than any other one. I got the job of massaging her daily to help her cope with the separation from her mother. I massaged her and gave her the bottle; and because I did not belong to the regular staff I was able to take my time.

Despite the fact that the baby was gaining weight, I felt that something was not quite right. She did not maintain eye contact, whenever I looked at her she looked away. I gave her massages and baths in daily rhythm, which she seemed to enjoy (rhythm builds trust and gives a feeling of security). After three days I noticed a change: the girl began to look into my eyes and hold my gaze. We had started a relationship! And despite the fact that outwardly there was no change, I felt that something important had happened. For the first time the same person had appeared day after day and she could dare to start a connection. This child was very well looked after and had got a lot of attention. It also had rhythm in its daily occurrences — but the personal environment lacked continuity and reliability and there was no regular connection person.

Then I started to think about what effect it would have on the baby if I also disappeared out of her life after she had dared to trust me. But we were lucky: on the day of my departure the grandmother came and took the baby home.

This necessity for a regular person is an important argument for involving the mother in the care of hospitalized infants.

### The role of the senses in the bonding process

Bonding can only happen with the help of the senses. They are the bridge between the emotional life and the outer world and other people, and we use all of them when we engage with a child.

### The eyes

Our eyes cannot lie. They show our feelings. The child is dependant on the love, care and joy that shines out of our eyes when we look after it or play with it.

### The sense of smell

The sense of smell is well developed in newborns, and they react strongly to different smells. They can identify their mother and find her breast with the help of smelling. Odent found that babies had difficulties finding the nipple when there were strong smells in the room.[12]

### Hearing

Long before birth the baby can hear sounds from the outside world. Pregnant women tell how their unborn babies react noticeably to music, and more than one mother has told me that they had to leave loud rock concerts because their babies were protesting with continued, extreme kicking.[13]

Speech plays an elemental part in the bonding process. Feelings like impatience and joy resound in our voice. Infants can hear our love and astonishment and admiration. They can understand exactly what we say — not the words themselves but their deeper meaning.

Without language we are isolated from other people. The well-known experiment by the German Emperor, Frederick II (1194–1250) shows how this can literally be deadly:

> He wanted to find out what language children learn and how they speak if they grow up without anybody talking to them. He told the wet-nurses to feed, bathe and clothe them without talking to them. He hoped to find out if the children would learn the ancient languages Hebrew, Latin or Greek, or the language of their parents. But his experiment failed: all the children died. They could not live without the loving attention and speech of their carers. That is why singing lullabies is so important.[14]

It is interesting that infants react especially to the higher frequency of women's voices, and that in all cultures women make their voices higher when speaking to babies.

### Taste

The sense of taste is extremely well developed in small children. Our sense of taste is actually there to help choose our food, but we spoil the taste buds of our children early on with our

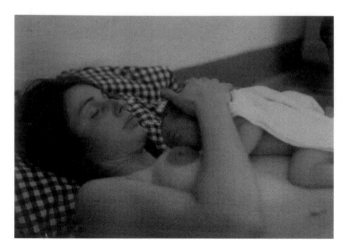

'civilized' food — artificial flavours, preservatives etc. We end up having to read books about nutrition, which then further confuse us because every expert says something different. But Nature has given us our instincts to rely on, if we do not blunt them by unnatural excess.

Breast milk is the best food, even vitamin-enhanced milk powder does not change that fact. This fact is generally accepted nowadays, unlike in the '50s and '60s, when mothers were totally confused. As well as all the physiological advantages of breast milk, such as immunization against certain illnesses, the connection between mother and child becomes even stronger through breastfeeding.

## Sense of balance

I want to mention the sense of balance which is so important for our development. The vestibular system — the sense of balance in the ear — is responsible for orientation in space. We have probably all experimented with it as children, when we twirled around until we fell down.

It seems that stimulating the vestibular system in the infant by rocking and rhythmical movement improves neurological development. There are hardly any nations that do not support this development in some way: whether through rocking, carrying, hammocks etc. We have got rid of the cradle as part of "progress" in the West because it is old-fashioned and we do not want to "spoil" our children.[15] What a difference from other nations. I lived in Africa for a long time and was fascinated by how naturally mothers carried their children on their backs — even when they were washing clothes in the river. Every time they bent over to submerge a piece of washing the child was tipped upside down for a moment.

Why are we afraid of spoiling our children if we carry them around? This is often discussed in antenatal classes and massage courses. People are still insecure. We do not seem to be able to tell the difference between a wrong concession, a let-anything-happen attitude, and real warmth and gentleness, but where you can still say an appropriate 'no.'

> *You cannot spoil a child through rocking,*
> *carrying and gentleness*

# The skin

When we say 'loving licking', or tactile stimulation of the skin, we are talking not only about the important point of affection, but also about the healthy organic development of every living creature...[16]

## *The importance of tactile stimulation for newborns*

Baby massage is described in detail in the second part of this book as I think this is one of the best ways of fulfilling the basic need for touch. In Western civilization we have repressed the knowledge of how elementary and biologically necessary touch is, which probably also results from the church's teaching that the body and bodily contact are sinful. Bodily pleasures and sensuality were synonymous with destruction and the fall from paradise. But we have also found that the general sense of promiscuity since the '60s did not satisfy in the long run. Hundreds of years of suppression disrupting our connection to our body and sexuality cannot be briefly healed by a radically opposite approach. The solution needs to be an inner process of liberation. Only once we are free of inhibitions, guilt and the confines of our upbringing and have achieved a loving relationship with our body will we be able to freely enjoy our sexuality. At this point we will make healthy choices and enter relationships that nourish and advance us. The fact that the West has a compulsive obsession with sex and a flourishing pornography industry is not a good sign, but rather proof that we lack access to a fulfilling, enriching sexuality.

Most of us have to learn to enjoy sensuality without inner restraint. Possibly gentleness and sensuality have got lost because we were not touched and caressed enough as babies.

The skin is not only necessary for the bonding process and thus for our social behaviour and psychological development, but also for bodily functions and growth. We can see by the behaviour of animals how important stimulating the skin is. Animals lick their young as feeding alone is not enough for survival. If the mother stops licking for any reason her young will die, because the urogenital system cannot function without the skin being stimulated.

There are hardly any nations that lick their babies — with the exception of polar regions and Tibet, where babies are sometimes cleaned in this way due to lack of water. Montagu states that the hours of labour in humans replaces the licking after birth.

Mothers who do not suffer from serious problems and who still have a healthy instinct automatically stroke, hold and caress their babies.

The skin envelops us entirely, it is the organ that develops first, it is our first means of exchange and our most effective protection. Apart from the brain it is probably the most important of our organic systems. The sense of touch, connected directly to the skin, is the source of our feelings, the first of the senses to develop in an embryo. It is a general rule of embryo development that the earlier a function develops, the more important it is.[17]

Massage is a good way of satisfying this need. It not only supports the organism in all its functions, but also gives the touch that skin requires. And — more importantly — the child experiences security and attention, and develops trust and confidence.

Massage is one of the best ways to help patients (children and adults) both physically and psychologically. It not only supports the functions of the organs, but advances a sense of well-being in general. Loosening tensions in the body can bring parallel relief on a psychological level. Feelings of fear and loneliness are dissipated by the individual attention. The following words of Dr Frederick Leboyer are probably his most frequently quoted:

We need to feed and overfeed them,
with warmth and gentleness.
Because they need it
as much as they need milk.

To be touched, caressed, massaged
that is nourishment for the child.

Nourishment which is as important
as minerals, vitamins, proteins,
nourishment which is love.
If a child is forced to do without,
it would rather die.
And often it really does die.[18]

The next chapter deals with early development and describes scientific evidence about the effect of tactile stimulation on the physiological processes of the body. We will see how bodily stimulation can release feelings and how these help determine the chemical and hormonal processes in the body.

The following pages about physiology are not so important for treating the child, rather they contain interesting research information scientifically proving the importance of the way we treat our babies.

If you want to treat a child directly and do not have enough time to read about theoretical background you can go straight to page 39, "Basic Principles of Massage." There you will find suggestions on how to give the child what it needs most and how to easily but effectively support it during medical treatment. To practically help your child you do not need to read the chapter about physiological processes.

# II. Development and Physiology

## Brain development

### *Why experiences in the first six months are so important*

The human being is actually born prematurely so that its head can fit through the narrow birth canal. It enters the world in an underdeveloped state and needs longer to become independent than other mammals. But it is not an advantage to remain longer in the uterus: perinatal death rates in overdue babies are double those of babies born on time.

> The gestation (Latin: carrying) does not end at birth, but continues beyond. Thus we have uterogestation (carrying in the uterus) and exterogestation (carrying outside the uterus). Bostock suggested exterogestation lasts until the child can crawl... It is interesting that the average exterogestation takes about $266^{1}/_{2}$ days, exactly as long as the pregnancy.[19]

### *Brain Growth Spurt Period*

The brain develops in two phases:
1. Between the 10th and approximately the 18th week of pregnancy the adult quantity of nerves has formed.
2. From the 18th to the 20th week of pregnancy until the second year of life the nerves grow and mature. This second phase is called the brain growth period. The brain is not fully developed at birth and still needs to mature. The process does not happen gradually but in growth spurts.

### *Weight of the brain*

> *The greatest brain growth is during the first six months of life*

— At birth 25% of adult weight.
— After six months 50% of adult weight[20]

The brain circumference of the child at its third birthday is already 90% of the adult brain and will only change insignificantly (Montagu).

### *The brain in the first half-year*

Brain researchers have found that the first six months are an extremely sensitive growth period. The greatest neurological development occurs and the foundations are laid for the rest of life. Physiological and psychological research has shown how impressionable the brain is during the first six months.

Lack of touch and attention during this sensitive phase of brain development is especially damaging. If we cannot fulfil the needs of the child in the first six months we can expect psychological disturbances in later life. These following problems can occur:

— depression
— feelings of loneliness
— self-hatred
— lack of confidence
— incapability of maintaining long-term relationships later in life
— the feeling of not being in control of life and not coping with stress
— irrational fears
— guilt with no apparent cause
— aggression

Katherine Asper believes estrangement from the self may be another consequence of early disturbances. Since their self-awareness is hazy these people have difficulties in finding a true identity, never quite getting a clear feeling as to who they really are. They therefore have difficulties with boundaries, are easily influenced or manipulated and find it hard to fend for themselves.

## Our chance to help

> *Damage done during this crucial time of neurological development is more serious and takes longer to heal than deprivation or trauma experienced later in life*

The vulnerability of the immature nervous system and the resulting impressionability also give us the chance to encourage the development of the child during this early phase. Enjoyable experiences, loving attention and bodily contact leave as lasting impressions as negative experiences. This means we have the chance to help and heal problems like premature birth, impaired growth, traumas, sleeping problems etc. with intensive gentle, bodily contact and regular tactile stimulation.

By giving regular and consistent treatment during the first two to three years of life, i.e. before brain growth is completed, growth retardation at birth may be compensated.

Dobbing and Dr Rice claim that tactile and muscular stimulation further neurological development. This view is supported by different studies. In these studies the greatest differences from the control groups, in the area of neurological development, were the massaged premature babies.

*The effect of tactile stimulation on neurological development:*

— more complexity of the dendrites (branched 'conductor' that transfer excitement between the nerve cells)
— increase of the myelin sheath (insulating sheath of the nerves)
— less production of adrenaline (stress hormone)
— general better endocrine (hormonal) function

Surely these scientific results are a motivation for anyone working with babies.

# Physiology

Happiness is the antidote to aggression.

## *Effect of tactile stimulation on the hormonal system*

### *The limbic system — ACTH and STH*

The drawing below shows a cross-section of the human brain with a simplified schematic depiction of the limbic system (arrows). The limbic system is like a switch between the perceptions of the sensory organs and the processes in the endocrine system.

It controls affective behaviour and impulses and their connection with the vegetative organ functions, and it is probably also important for memory.

### *Limbic system and feelings*

Afferent nerves — the nerve paths leading towards the brain — conduct stimulations from the periphery to the spinal cord, and from there to the brain, which means that all sensory perceptions — from the eyes, ears, skin, smell and taste organs — are transferred to the brain and then to the limbic system. Once there the stimulations received from the sensory organs are evaluated as feelings. Impressions from the outside world are experienced as either pleasant or unpleasant sensations. Nerve and chemical stimulation become feelings! The limbic system directs the way we react to stimulation and strongly influences our well-being as well as our social and sexual behaviour.

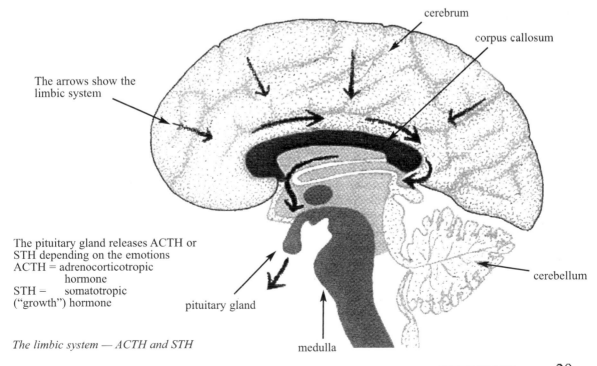

The arrows show the limbic system

cerebrum

corpus callosum

cerebellum

The pituitary gland releases ACTH or STH depending on the emotions
ACTH = adrenocorticotropic hormone
STH = somatotropic ("growth") hormone

pituitary gland

medulla

*The limbic system — ACTH and STH*

Chemically the limbic system has a direct connection with the hypothalamus, the higher regulatory organ of the hormones. The hypothalamus regulates the pituitary gland and dictates which hormones are released into the blood (see diagram).

> *The material and the emotional meet*
> *in the limbic system*

## Limbic system and memory

The limbic system also seems to be important for the retention of experiences, although it is not yet quite clear in what way. Psychology has taught us that none of our experiences are lost. Situations accompanied by strong emotions leave particularly deep impressions and are never forgotten. They often unconsciously determine our behaviour even late in life.

> *Feelings like well-being, fear, stress and joy affect*
> *the endocrine system. It means they influence the*
> *hormonal composition of the blood and thus the physi-*
> *ological processes, the immune system and growth!*

## Hormones and feelings

### Continual stress and resignation — "inhibition of action syndrome"

Incubators and intensive care are extremely distressing for a baby, both physically and psychologically. The sensory organs are overstimulated. Bright light and loud noises surround the child, which lies motionless and isolated without bodily contact in the incubator. Most of the touches the child experiences are of a painful nature; infusions, injections and blood samples. Thus a dangerous vicious circle can develop if a newborn has to remain in this situation for days or even weeks.

The body prepares for fight or flight in extreme stress situations by producing noradrenaline. The child can neither resist its situation nor flee. Noradrenaline activates the hypothalamus and keeps it in an excited state. The body produces cortisone which stops movement and reactions. As a result the pathological condition "inhibition of action" ensues. The child gives up and surrenders to its hopeless situation. It remains apathetic even when subjected to painful procedures and does not even react by crying. This reaction has led to the belief that newborns do not feel pain.

As we have seen, feelings are important in the early developmental phase. Deprivation, loneliness, physical and emotional injuries of any kind influence our behaviour, leading to completely inadequate and "emotional" reactions to some situations. This in turn leads to the development of behavioural patterns. When memories of difficult experiences are triggered in certain circumstances they then control our behaviour. We react to them as if they were the original distress and assess the now harmless situation unrealistically — as if we were in real danger. As this is an unconscious process neither our intelligence nor reasoning helps. We are flooded with emotions, for example unwarranted jealousy, irrational fear and fantasies. Our body also responds with a faster heartbeat, heavy breathing etc.

I know this from my own experience: I spent the first years of my life in Germany, the second World War had just started when I was born. My first memories are of endless nights spent in bunkers, bomb alerts, continuous danger and frightened adults, who were so worried they had hardly any time to look after us children. Many years later, when I was already living in Switzerland, I woke up at night sweating and with my heart pounding whenever I heard certain types of aeroplane flying overhead. I was already over forty years old, but my biological memory still registered alarm whenever I heard that noise. When I realized where the panic came from and established the connection with the war these attacks stopped. But my pulse still quickens whenever I hear those aeroplanes. The faster, much louder jets of today's airforce do not cause any reaction — they did not exist in those days and are not connected in my subconscious to my early childhood death fears. Thus I can react *sensibly* and assess whether there is real danger or not.

Such patterns of behaviour influence us all more or less strongly. The less we are conscious of them, the more power they have over us, for example in our relationships and jobs. They block a lot of energy, rob us of spontaneity and prevent us from developing our unique personality to its full potential.

Working through early childhood wounds makes us more liberated.

## The endocrine system

Science describes how our well-being or stress influences our endocrine system, and thus our hormones. Everett W. Bovard found that stroking ("handling") rats right after birth heightened the pituitary/adrenal reactions.[21] This shows that gentle stroking changes the content of the hormonal balance to such an extent that we can become calmer, healthier and more balanced, and develop a thicker "skin" against stress, whether physical or psychological.

Bovard stresses the fact that continuous, extended irritation and excitement attack kidneys, heart and circulation. Our lifestyle continually overstimulates the senses and nerves, leading to illnesses as a result of 'civilization' like heart-circulation problems, diabetes and rheumatism.

And this is what your hormonal balance looks like.

| *Well-being and relaxation excite the parasympatheticum* | | *Fear and stress excite the sympatheticum* | |
|---|---|---|---|
| STH = growth hormone | + | adrenocortical hormone | + |
| Stress hormone | – | Adrenaline (stress hormone) | + |
| Heart beat | – | Heart beat | + |
| Oxygen consumption | – | Oxygen consumption | + |
| Coherence of brain halves (increased intelligence) | + | Blood pressure | + |
| Alpha waves | + | | |

If a baby is stroked lovingly more growth hormones are released into the blood. Dr Rice's research shows that massaged babies have faster growth and weight gain.

The amount of oxygen the body uses shows how stressed the organism is. When relaxed the amount of oxygen needed decreases by 10%–20% in the first three minutes, which helps regeneration and recovery.

In a relaxed state both sides of the brain work together more efficiently. This not only increases our intelligence, but gives us better access to our abilities and intuition. It becomes easier for us to express our creative potential.

If our brain produces alpha waves we experience a feeling of calm and peace. These alpha waves can be measured with modern machines. More and more people use methods like deep relaxation and meditation to revive, experience peace and joy and release their potential energy and talents.

## The immune system

The body acquires an increased ability to ward off illnesses when it is treated. While stress hormones damage the body, feeling good strengthens it. Most of us know this from our own experience. If we are engaged in an important task that we enjoy, if we are needed or have even fallen in love, then everybody around us can get flu while we remain healthy. If for some reason we are depressed or suffer from stress or lack of sleep then we will soon join our sick colleagues. It is not the virus that causes illness, but the condition of our organism and its inability to cope with attacks. A strengthened body and a happy nature are best for staving off viruses and bacteria.

Here is a conclusion from psychosomatic research, cited in the book *The Guide to Child Health:*

> Psychoneuroimmunological research has confirmed that positive emotions like courage, enthusiasm, trust and love stimulate the human immune system while stress, anger, fear, lethargy and depression weaken it.[22]

Tension decreases when basic needs are met. Research shows that where there is joy there cannot be stress, fear or aggression. Well-being and security are a most effective treatment. They change the hormonal composition of the blood, and thus enhance physical and psychological development and strengthen the immune system. Such findings show that we can do something to increase the resistance of children prone to infections. Admittedly, loving touch and other natural remedies appear too simple to help the confusing and complex problems that confront us. But never underestimate simple things! We desperately need them. One cannot deny that despite impressive surgical improvements and treatments of a few infectious diseases children's health is deteriorating continuously. Children's susceptibility to illnesses is a great worry. European doctors urge us to take action, as breathing difficulties and lung diseases in small children have risen alarmingly. Some reports say that allergies in the population have increased fourfold in just one generation. Childhood illnesses develop atypically and have become difficult to diagnose. Drug resistant bacteria cannot be fought with antibiotics.

While writing this chapter I have coincidentally received an article from the *Sunday Telegraph* called "Invasion of the superbugs."[23] The article describes a new publication: Geoffrey Cannon, *Superbug, Nature's revenge*. The book is a warning against the misuse of antibiotics:

> Wisely used antibiotics are a blessing. But they are now vastly overused and abused. The US National Institute of Health has estimated that by the year 2000, a total of 50,000 tons will be used every year throughout the world on humans, animals and plants, amoutning to a vast, unplanned, unchecked and uncontrollable exercise in bacterial genetic manipulation. The scale of use makes mass microbial mutation, and with it new forms of disease, inevitable.

The following explanation given by Geoffrey Cannon should make us think twice about using antibiotics:

> We have been brought up to believe that bacteria are generally harmful, and to confuse hygiene with sterility. This is a mistake. We need the bugs that live on and in us; almost all of them have evolved to be harmless or positively health-giving to their host, whether human, animal or plant.
>
> Among other functions, harmless bacteria protect us against invasive infection simply by being there. The bacteria in our guts, sometimes known as friendly flora, amount to a vital organ of our body.
>
> There is no such thing as a magic bullet, meaning a drug whose one and only effect is to destroy disease. Exactly like pesticides, antibiotics make waves in the ecosphere. The more they are used, and the more broad-spectrum they are in their effect, the more bacterial species they devastate, creating a microbiological wasteland. This is liable to be invaded and colonised by other bacterial species, some originally harmless, others essentially harmful, and also by moulds, viruses and other microbes, which may cause what is known as superinfectious disease.*
>
> Heavy or regular use of some antibiotics, liable to damage the mucosal lining of the gut wall and thus our immune defences, is for this, and other reasons, possibly one cause of a number of diseases that baffle modern medical science, some much more common in the last half century. These include gut diseases such as irritable bowel syndrome and perhaps even colon cancer, some forms of arthritis and the debilitating illness known as chronic fatigue syndrome or ME.
>
> The intestines of people who take antibiotics are factories producing drug-resistant bacteria.[24]

We are slowly realizing that the dream of the fifties, that every illness would soon be under control, is an illusion. The huge, nearly euphoric belief in science and technology is being hit by disappointments. As a consequence we do not embrace nor accept unconditionally every new scientific finding. This means everyone is faced with huge new challenges. While scientists and doctors argue

---

* Superinfection is a re-infection by the same germ during the initial infection before the body has acquired immunity.

against each other, mothers and fathers have to make important decisions. They need to decide, for example, which vaccination is or is not beneficial, or if a prescribed antibiotic treatment is really necessary. Since they receive conflicting evidence from professionals, parents need to inform themselves, weigh up the risks and make their own decisions. Choosing a doctor needs careful consideration, as he or she should understand and support the parents' individual life philosophy.

The lack of trust in science necessitates the greater responsibility of every individual. Doctors have to become less of an authority and more a companion during the process. The expectation that every illness can be controlled and cured by vaccinations and chemicals leads to an unrealistic approach to health. Through losing these illusions we are forced to take responsibility for our own health — and its connection to habit and lifestyle — rather than blaming doctors and hospitals for our illnesses. The increasing willingness to take part in improving our health is mirrored in the growing interest in natural remedies and healthy eating.

# Development and violence

How poor is our life, if nothing in us is immortal.[25]

We know from developmental psychology that babies who lack touch and attention are more inclined towards violence as an adult. Contented, "satisfied" babies whose basic needs are fulfilled would thus be the best prevention against the increase in violence in our society. Many people have problems accepting the importance of this statement, saying it is part of human nature to be violent and there have always been wars — peace is an illusion. This is how "realists" argue, and history appears to support their views. Underneath this pessimistic prognosis lies a perception of humanity that does not believe in individual or collective development. The current position of things is perceived as an unchangeable fact of fate and not as a phase of a spiritual, developmental process. Thus the theme of violence is seen as a political problem, and politicians blame it on the high unemployment rate and the lack of equal education opportunities.

However, stopping violence does not begin with the state or a research centre, but in the individual soul. Whether we believe it or not, every one of us affects the whole of the world, as there is no separation in nature and nobody can exist alone. What concerns one person concerns everybody.

In one of the popular phenomenon-exhibitions in Zurich this fact was demonstrated by an experiment. A few hundred 6–7 cm high little sticks that could move horizontally in any direction, were attached above a table. They were loosely connected to each other, and could be moved in different patterns and rhythms by jolting the table. If one only moved one of these sticks (which looked like people standing in a row) by touching it gently with a finger to change the direction of its "dance," then the whole group began to move in a different way. A small change of an individual stick influenced the behaviour of them all! This law works in all areas of human living – and in the whole cosmos.

It is not an exaggeration to say that every happy and content person contributes to world peace. Peace starts with each individual. And probably the biggest contribution to a peaceful future are children who have grown up happy. If we understand the causes of aggressive behaviour better, then we are also able to find an effective treatment. Violence is not necessary. It does not inevitably belong to our nature. We need to believe in our power to change things and in our ability to create peace.

## Possible reasons for aggressive behaviour

| Early childhood disturbance through deprivation | psychological pain |
| --- | --- |
| Wrong diet | bodily pain |
| Lack of meaning in life | mental pain |

### Early childhood deprivation
Plenty of bodily contact, gentle touch and emotional attention at an early age prepare against later aggressive and violent behaviour. Research accounts supporting this have been available for years.[26] Whoever has experienced that they are loveable and have a healthy self-esteem can react to frustrations encountered in life in a different way than violently or aggressively. We have seen that joy and aggression are in opposition. Wherever there is happiness there is no space for aggression and violence. Inadequacy, whether of a physical or psychological nature, make us dissatisfied and angry, feelings that can overshadow everything else in later life. For some unexplained reason we never feel quite comfortable. Later we are not able to stick up for ourselves and feel helpless, or we react in some situations with disproportionately strong emotions and violence.

### The wrong diet causes aggression

The character of our children is not only a matter of inheritance and upbringing but a large part of it is determined through our diet. The fact that there could be a connection between diet and aggressive behaviour is still not given enough attention in medical circles. But diet is one of the most important factors that determine our behaviour. The current overfeeding of calories and at the same time the lack of vital substances overburden our metabolism and immune system. This disturbs the equilibrium of our organism and harms our health. If the body is lacking necessary substances for important functions then our sense of life is affected and we suffer from apathy, fatigue and lack of enthusiasm,. We become 'acidic,' because our body's acid-alkaline equilibrium has been disrupted. We become tearful, overstrung and aggressive.

Dr Lothar Burgerstein dedicates a whole chapter in his book to diet and criminality.

There is no doubt that besides social conditions bad diet and too much sugar contributes to the increasing aggression of youths. Young people consume a lot of sweet food and drinks and often eat fast food.[27]

Burgerstein, who has contributed a lot towards spreading orthomolecular medicine in Switzerland describes how American jails and reformatories have shown great success by changing their diet.* He introduces the work of Alex G. Schauss.[28]

According to him, forty-two of the fifty American states are dealing with the connection between food and crimes, and conducting practical tests with a high success rate. The change in diet especially relates to sugar content and factory-produced fast food. Sugar has been banned from the menu wherever possible, soft drinks have been substituted by fruit juices, tinned food by fresh food. The well-being and behaviour of the inmates has changed positively since introducing this new nutrition.

High meat consumption is also not without problems for more than one reason. Apart from the fact that meat production is an environmental problem, eating meat in such great amounts is bad for our health. Animal proteins are difficult to digest and make the organism too acidic. Cattle are treated with antibiotics while being reared. When the animal is brought to be slaughtered, it produces stress and fear hormones, and its adrenaline level rises dramatically. These elements are all later ingested.

Research shows increasingly that there is a correlation between disturbed behaviour, youth criminality, vandalism etc. and food. Herta Hafner has looked at the effect of food containing phosphate on the behaviour of hyperactive children and discusses the connections in her book.[29] These investigations also showed that changing the diet of phosphate-sensitive children brought a marked improvement in their symptoms. A good diet currently requires a lot more consciousness, attention and discipline.

The BBC ran a remarkable news item that stated that the seagulls in a popular English holiday resort were becoming increasingly aggressive, attacking people, particularly their heads, and injuring them with their sharp beaks.[30] There were so many instances of this happening that the council decided to shoot the violent birds. Interestingly, the councillors felt that the tourists were causing the attacks by feeding the birds junk food. Chips, hamburgers and other fast food appeared to be the reason for the aggression.

An involuntary experiment on animals! In this case the connection between food and aggression was noticed straight away. But this awareness is lacking when it comes to ourselves or our children. Sooner or later the connection will become clear. Wrong, unnatural food also makes the soul ill.

## Lack of meaning in life causes aggression

A person is impoverished without a spiritual goal. The general increased lack of enthusiasm and discontentment is the product of a lack of

---

* Orthomolecular medicine describes the practice of preventing and treating disease by providing the body with optimal amounts of substances which are natural to the body (www.orthomed.org)

direction in life. Our culture is so geared towards material values and consumption, and the education system so geared towards the intellect, that we are becoming increasingly impoverished. All public decisions are discussed and decided upon from a material point of view. Spiritual and religious values are pushed to the side and regarded with disdain for being unrealistic and unscientific. Prayer has virtually been abandoned in schools. In contrast to other cultures we separate religion completely from public living. Religious feelings are well hidden and held privately, as if they are shameful. Who can still imagine starting a business meeting with a prayer?

But life means growth, and the laws of evolution push people to search for spiritual values and metaphysical experiences. Humans look for a deep, personal, 'Godly' experience that remains their own, and carries and accompanies them through all difficulties. This longing is planted deeply in everyone. Not even the greatest riches will silence it, and if it is repressed and remains in the unconscious, it causes all sorts of problems, for example aggression, unhappiness or flight into drugs. Often it is sensitive and vulnerable young people who are drawn to drugs because they cannot cope with the senseless emptiness of the prevailing superficiality around them.

The generation of young people who have just grown up in Western industrial countries have experienced a level of wealth previously unknown. The social state, fought for by the great thinkers and statesmen since the beginning of the industrial revolution, has been expanded in every detail. I have spent most of my life in Switzerland, the country with probably the most wealth. People buying the newest things and needing to throw away so much has led to a huge problem of getting rid of rubbish. But where are all the contented people? Where is the happy society we were promised when unemployment and material misery were eliminated?

Our young people suffer from yawning boredom despite television and computer games. Every child shows us: 'we do not live by bread alone.' But nothing points towards us having understood it. Not in public life, nor in governments or institutions do we take the law into account. Even churches have mainly become social establishments, which look after the poor, ill and excluded. Where is the fire, the life joy, the courage that stems from the knowledge that the material world is transient and we are spiritual beings, able to draw from unlimited sources if we adhere to spiritual laws?

Meeting a place of permanence and godliness in our own soul brings great calmness and joy. A society that disregards spiritual values destroys itself. Whoever experiences themselves as part of an organization spanning all things is religious. Being religious means experiencing that the deepest, most intimate part of oneself is at the same time part of the cosmos. This is where mature behaviour starts, taking on both the responsibility for personal deeds and the needs of the collective. Aggression and fear disappears.

The brutal reality of the so-called realists is not an inevitable fate. Rather, we continually construct our reality and fate through the priorities we set. As we think, so we become. We create our conditions ourselves, and they are changeable through reforming our inner values. The only thing that probably remains unchangeable in our so-called reality are the spiritual laws governing everything.

# Knowledge which leads to actions

Newspaper articles, literature and research papers show how much we theoretically know about children's development at the moment. But being informed does not mean being able to understand or grasp the matter. Information from research is only meaningful if we also follow the findings. At a lecture held at a conference "giving birth safely and with confidence" (Zurich, 1992), Dr Michael Odent remarked about birthing practices and the way we treat babies:

> Never before has the gap been so great between what studies have researched and recognized, and what we effectively do.[31]

The discrepancy between knowing and doing is a lack of connection between the head and the heart. We read a lot, are overwhelmed with a mass of media information, and our "knowledge" of birth and children could fill libraries. But we can really only speak of real knowledge when the information has become internalized, influencing our daily life and improving our quality of life. The word "grasp" means both to understand something and to hold, grip and touch something. What we have grasped we have understood with our feelings and with our sensory organs, not just in an abstract way with our intellect. It is only then that information becomes a useful enrichment.

The gap that Odent talks about will not be closed by scientific research institutions or universities, but first and foremost in our consciousness and at the bedsides of individual patients. We need to have the courage to love.

While writing these thoughts I was reminded of a story that a relative told me many years ago. She was working in a district hospital on the paediatric ward. The clinic was reknowned because of a professor who was an expert in his area and was feared by the staff because of his strictness. One night a nurse heard a voice coming out of one of the rooms. The door was open slightly and as she neared it she saw the professor speaking encouragingly to a very ill child and rocking it in his arms.

An effective and simple way of bringing in a level of feeling into nursing is massaging and other methods of body treatment described below. They are logical, consistent transformations of our theoretical knowledge about the basic needs of humans.

Before explaining baby massage and the various other methods I want to describe the basis of body therapies. From my experience of treating adults and babies these basic rules are very important and only through observing them can technique be transformed into a form of art. You will soon notice that the effect of the body therapy is not so dependant on the method, but rather on your inner attitude, thoughts and feelings, attention and sensitivity. In the end it is you, with your whole personality and compassion, that brings the healing element into the technique, irrespective of the method you choose.

# III. Basic Principles of Massage

## Introduction

As with all natural treatments perseverance and regularity arc of prime importance for body treatments like polarity, massage and the RISS method. I always encourage parents and nursing staff to incorporate massage into the daily nursing routine and to set aside enough time for it. If you wait until you have enough time you will probably wait a long time. There always appear to be more pressing matters. Tasks incorporated into the daily rhythm are more likely to be enacted. This is true both at home and in hospital. Babies love rhythm, it gives them a sense of security.

Massage can be practised from birth onwards and is suitable for both healthy and sick children. You can massage for as long as the child is comfortable with being massaged, which varies from child to child. Some lose interest when they start to crawl, when they want to discover their surroundings rather than lie still. Often they show interest again at a later stage. Around the ages of three or four, children who are used to massage often demonstrate exactly what they want: touching their back, reciting verses while being massaged or stroking some part of their body.[32]

Claire Gauch shows how teenagers can also be receptive to massage in her book *Die Macht der Zärtlichkeit* (*The Power of Gentleness*).[33]

If asked up to which age it is suitable to massage babies I always tell a story that I heard from a therapist in New York: an old lady broke her thigh when she fell and needed to spend quite some time in hospital. Her children came to visit and noticed she had not looked so young and radiant for a long time. When they asked her the reason for this, the woman began to cry and said that in the hospital she had been touched by someone for the first time in fifteen years.

This story is a good answer to the question when we should stop touching or massaging each other. Being touched is a basic need and most people are happy to receive loving touch whatever their age. When working in old peoples' homes I always tried to complement washing with a massage. Usually it was only a few minutes of a back or foot massage, as the hospital's agenda did not include time for any more, but a few touches were always possible with the patients who enjoyed it. I was moved at their gratefulness for such a small gesture.

Since touching and being touched is a general human requirement I answer the often-asked question whether baby massage comes from India, with: "No, touch is actually international." The wish for gentle touch has nothing to do with country, culture or age. Therefore, tactile stimulation or "gentle touch" is suitable from birth — including premature or sick babies — until old age. The technique is adapted according to the circumstances (see the chapter on contra indications on page 88).

> *Tactile stimulation is suitable from birth — also for sick or premature babies.*

## The effect of massage on bodily processes

Whether we massage for pleasure, to prevent illness or as a therapy, the effect is always better if we massage regularly over a period of time. Apart from the previously described advantages to the development of the child and parental bonding, all bodily functions are supported and regulated. The nerves in different areas of the skin are closely connected with the internal organs, and thus in a position to affect them. Organs deep inside our body are stimulated by touch to the skin.

The following processes are directly influenced by massage:
— Blood supply and detoxification
— Breathing
— Digestion (children with colic should be massaged regularly!)
— Sleep
— Immunity (less prone to infections)

A massage harmonizes the whole organism and leaves us feeling relaxed and revitalized. Limp tissue becomes toned and muscles cramps are loosened. The following are a few instances where regular massage is worth trying:

— premature babies;
— caesarean babies (they receive a lot less tactile stimulation during birth than vaginal births);
— children with colic;
— children that always have colds or other breathing difficulties;
— babies that do not seem to thrive;
— children that do not sleep properly;
— hyperactive children;
— hypoactive children.

Healthy babies will profit just as much from a massage as sick ones will, and massage may even help to prevent some conditions. Why wait until your baby is ill? You could get into this beneficial habit now!

## Inner attitude

It is not the choice of method or the technique which governs the effectiveness of treatment, but the attention and inner attitude of the person giving treatment.

Treating a body is the same as practising music, the musician needs to know his instrument and be in command of technique. However, the audience is not touched by technical ability, but by artistic expression. An artwork is created by the unique and personal interpretation of the artist which comes from the artist's innermost core.

It is the same for massage. We learn different techniques and strokes, but massage becomes an artform when we work from our inner self using our attentiveness and joy. If we do not give anything of ourselves to the treatment it remains cold and the effect is minimal. The inner attitude and connection with other people are more important than method and technique. A masseur that works indifferently or mechanically turns a massage into an exercise. For real treatment completely different qualities are needed from merely rehearsed techniques. Complete attention and concentration are required. It is not possible to remain in this state of awareness while chatting to someone else.

### Inner attitude during treatment

Authenticity and honesty are necessary requirements for treating. No patient or child will be fooled by a sweet voice if there is no real participation behind it. Make sure the things you do correspond to what you feel and think, otherwise they harm more than they help. Our hands cannot lie. A child receives a confusing message if you treat it without inner conviction. Although it is stroked by your hands, its feelings receive a different message. Thus it is very important to observe and be aware of your feelings. We are not always in a loving and caring mood. We do not automatically love our patients and children. Most of us experience negative feelings towards our babies when responsibility overwhelms us, we are worried or our freedom is curtailed, especially if our needs as a baby were not met. However, we can learn to develop by taking ourselves and our feelings seriously, and trying to find out more about them. It is unconscious deeds and repressed feelings that are harmful.

These rules should be applied to any kind of

> *Our deeds should be honest —*
> *in agreement with our thoughts and feelings.*

interaction between people, but particularly in relationships with children and patients. As an educator or therapist we are in a position of power. The child deserves to be taken seriously. I think the following attitudes are a good prerequisite for treating adults as well as babies:

— no fixed ideas or expectations, never mind what happens
— high concentration and attention to everything that happens
— to be centred and calm
— unconditional acceptance of the other person
— no appraisal or judgement
— allow whatever happens to happen
— accompany the other person through their feelings and give them the chance to unburden themselves
— let go of compulsive and false 'comforting' by using different kinds of diversions
— work without trying to change the other person
— work without trying to 'achieve something!'

*Letting go of compulsive 'comforting': working through trauma and unburdening tensions.*

It is possible, even probable, that strong feelings are released by body therapy. Our body is a kind of life book that has its own memories. Our experiences, whether positive or negative, are stored in it. Early experiences with strong emotional content, or which are connected to survival, leave the deepest impression. Suppressing old wounds and unresolved traumas block our energy potential, spontaneity and creativity. On a bodily level these untreated wounds translate themselves into tense muscles, respiratory problems, circulatory problems etc. When we work with the body, it is possible that old traumas and experiences are re-activated with their intense emotions. Mental blocks originating in childhood slowly begin to dissolve. It is possible that deep pain, degradation and hurt are re-lived again.

It is important to let patients, whether children or adults, have so-called 'negative' outbursts like anger, fear, sadness and crying. As therapists we need an accepting, non-judgmental attitude, free from hidden agendas. When we have learnt to accept such feelings in ourselves our fellow human beings are also able to do so. People will notice if we do not fear strong emotion — ours or theirs — and will possibly let us accompany them along their way. This is what is meant by 'letting go of compulsive comforting.' It is often wrongly understood and interpreted as lack of compassion. Comforting in the usual sense is often an attempt to divert from pain, because we are incapable of coping with an outburst of emotion. However, someone who is sad or angry needs a person to notice and accept his feelings, not be diverted from them. Otherwise he will feel misunderstood.

There is a simple example of this: if a boy runs to his mother because he has fallen and grazed his knee, she can either accept his pain and say: "I see that is very painful," and hold him until he stops crying, and, if necessary, get a plaster, or she can react in a different way — and this is how most of us react — and say: "stop crying, it's not that bad." She not only gets a plaster, but also an ice cream from the freezer to stop him crying. The first reaction shows real sympathy and will leave a feeling of satisfaction. The second solution leaves an unpleasant feeling, and the 'comfort' is nothing but an attempt to distract. It is not surprising that the boy is left in a bad mood and tending to be naughty.

We also want to share our pain with someone else. It is not enough to grieve by ourselves, we need someone who can see our pain. I mention these situations because they shed light on an important theme, which applies not only to education but also to how we treat patients. As has been shown above the psychological state determines the physical processes to a large extent. If we do not attend to psychological needs the body cannot get better. Communicating strong emotions is the key to treating psychological wounds. We take note of the cause, and thus treat the whole person and not only the symptoms. We could save a huge amount in medicine and hospital beds if we took this fact into consideration when treating ill people.

If memories are evoked by massage or other types of physical treatment we have the opportunity to work through old traumas. The treatment is thus not only a procedure to loosen tension in the body, but also a healing aid for underlying psychological wounds.

The same principles hold true for baby massage. Babies are not always hungry or fed up with the massage when they cry, but possibly re-living a painful experience.[34] When working with a part of the body it is necessary to observe whether it could be connected with a bad experience. Babies, like adults, should not be diverted from their pain. Never leave the baby alone in such a situation. Hold it and give it the chance to finish crying even if you cannot see any reason for its grief or anger.

I was taught this by an incident with one particular mother. Nicole was forty when expecting her first child, and asked me to join her and her husband for the birth. It was a natural birth, but took a long time, and we used all sorts of methods to make the long first stage easier for Nicole. Between the three of us there was intense work and inspiration. I brought my tape recorder and the music appeared to be carrying Nicole. She danced and sang, and thus coped with the strongest labour pains. We were all very happy that Nicole and her baby managed the birth without a caesarean. This united experience of the birth left a deep connection and we stayed in contact. I heard from Nicole that Lukas cried a lot because of lower body pains, and had to be carried for hours on end. We arranged to meet for a baby massage. I massaged Lukas on the floor of the sitting room beside a stove. He obviously enjoyed being treated and was completely awake. At the end, though, he pulled a face and began to cry in a strange way. Straight away I went through the usual worries: was it too hot beside the stove, was he hungry, had I done something "wrong"? I tried to quieten him, but Nicole said: "You know, I think he just needs to cry a bit." She lifted him up and explained that it was fine for him to cry a bit, she understood that he was sometimes sad. Lukas cried for at least an hour. Sometimes his voice was angry, and his whole body convulsed and Nicole explained to him she could understand why he was angry. Sometimes his voice sounded sad and pensive — Nicole told him she was also sometimes sad. In between he stopped and looked his mother in the eyes. Then he continued screaming. Sometimes Nicole also cried, and once I also felt tears in my eyes, but in the end Lukas quietened. It was already late and the moon shone in the room. Lukas slept with a peaceful smile on his lips.

The 'meeting' had consequences. A few weeks later I heard that Lukas had changed since that evening. His digestive problems had practically vanished and he was much happier.

Sometimes connections are clearly visible. A mother came with her three-month-old daughter to be treated. The baby greatly enjoyed the massage, but when I touched her left shoulder, her whole body became tense and she held her arm against her body. When I asked the mother whether there had been any problems during the birth, she told me that there had been difficulties with that shoulder.

Sometimes I found that babies enjoyed the whole massage until I touched their heel. They then screamed inconsolably and protested against any further touch. It turned out that these babies had had their heel pricked for blood repeatedly after birth. The memory of these painful intrusions had been evoked by the touch. Such reactions can lead us to believe that the children do not like massage or that we have done something wrong. We should not give up too quickly under such circumstances.

## Effective help for old pains re-activated during massage

Old traumas brought into consciousness during treatment should be welcomed. Our reaction is important and determines the further course of treatment.

Depending on how we act, we can suppress, distract from, or help release, old pains. It would be a shame to discontinue massaging such a child. We should rather keep offering to work on those parts of the body that the child enjoys having massaged. If I know, for example, that the child reacts negatively to touch on their shoulder or foot, then I approach these areas with the utmost care, leave them out, or just lay my hand on the affected area until the child enjoys the touch and slowly forgets the old pains. A massage should never be forced.

The three-year-old daughter of a friend always made a fuss whenever she had shoes or socks put on. She did not want her feet touched. We started to hold her feet whenever we adults were talking, quietly and without making a big thing of it. I laid my hand without pressure around her foot, and once she had got used to that, I started to slowly and gently stroke it. She let it happen with her other foot as well, and after a few sessions she had got over her fear of being touched. The child had been premature and had spent a long time in intensive care.

The causes are not always so obvious, but healing through touch can happen even without a "diagnosis." I often experience a marked improvement even after only one massage treatment — as if a vicious circle is broken. A mother at the end of her tether came with her three-month-old son. She had not had a peaceful night since his birth, because he kept waking up at short intervals and crying without any obvious reason. The baby sighed deeply a few times as I massaged him, which is always a good sign of releasing tension (also in adult therapy). Afterwards the child appeared to be contented and relaxed. A few weeks later I heard that he had slept through the night for the first time after that treatment, and since then had only woken occasionally at night.

There are various things that indicate tension release.

> *Yawning, sighing, crying, giggling, shrieking and thrashing about can all be signs that the patient is releasing tension.*

The principle of releasing tension is extremely important. We cannot assume that the child does not like the treatment just because it is crying. Believe that it is good for the patient to be touched by your hands and that it is helpful if the child (or adult) cries during treatment, because old wounds are brought to the fore and released. Accompanying someone through pain is an effective therapy.

However we are only able to do this if we are ready to allow pain in ourselves, and can only accompany people to places we have dared to go ourselves.

> *We can only heal to the extent that we have allowed healing to happen in ourselves.*

The above is significant and if adhered to changes our style of upbringing and how we work with patients. Interest and honesty with regard to the process of self-development are prerequisites to gaining this level of depth in therapy.

# Preparation before treatment

Where all actions cease and silence prevails, light begins to flow.

## Inner preparation

An artist inevitably reveals his internal state through his work. It determines the themes and colours he chooses and his brushstroke. The same is true for massage. Treatment is more pleasurable and effective when done with inner peacefulness and concentration, but peacefulness and quietness do not come naturally to most of us. Life has too many distractions and problems. In addition, a lot of willpower is necessary to disconnect consciously from the frenzied and hectic lifestyle so typical of our time. However, becoming peaceful is a matter of practise. Whoever strives towards it will soon find that everyday duties become easier. Inner peace transfers itself to everything we undertake. I notice a difference in my treatments if I have been very busy for a few days before and unable to switch off and experience quiet.

Being relaxed and calm does not happen by demand. Certain techniques and aids are necessary to quieten a mood. There are many books and courses on this subject, and the key is to find one that suits your temperament. One technique I find very effective is *practising attentiveness*. I try to consciously direct my attention to different levels of the person — from the body through feelings to thoughts.

## Practising attentiveness

This is a classic yoga relaxation technique. Sit comfortably, but upright, in a chair. Investigate whether your shoulders are relaxed despite your straight spine. Hands should be on your thighs or in your lap. Feet should be firmly and flatly on the floor (no high heels!).

— Breathe in and out deeply a few times. Shut your eyes.
— Your whole attention should be on what is happening to yourself at this moment; how you feel there in your room, how you are sitting. Try and consciously observe how your body feels, with an attitude of complete acceptance and without judgement.
— Start with your feet. Feel the contact with the ground, the pressure of gravity, the whole sole of your foot, every single toe, the spaces between the toes, the arch of your foot, the ankle.
— With great concentration work your way up your body. Let your consciousness take note of everything like a inquisitive, interested observer (always without judging!).
— The shins, knees, thighs.
— The genitals and posterior, the pelvis, stomach and chest.
— The spine, each single vertebra from bottom to top, the whole back, the shoulders.
— Observe your hands: how are they placed? What are they touching? Feel every finger, the palms, the backs of the hand, the wrists.
— The forearms, elbows, upper arms, armpits, shoulders.
— Feel your neck, scalp, chin, teeth, gums, lips, cheeks, nose, nose tip, eyes and

eyelids. Feel how the eyelids gently touch the eyes.

— The eyebrows and forehead, the mid-point between your eyebrows. Keep bringing your attention back to your body if your mind wanders. Remain a neutral observer.

— Occupy your mind by concentrating on your breathing without interfering or manipulating it. Observe how your body moves with every breath, how there are small breaks between breathing in and out.

— Pay attention to your feelings, your mood. Take an inner step back and observe your feelings, accept them without becoming involved with them.

— Observe how your thoughts come and go continuously in wild sequence. Do not become too involved. Be an observer. Let your thoughts pass by, then come back to the present: your body, your breathing.

— Remain for a few more minutes in your position, experience how your breath flows through your body. Imagine you have become extensive and penetrable, your breath nourishing every cell of your body.

— Come back slowly to the outer word. Take a few deep breaths and stretch, refreshed for new tasks.

The more you practise, the easier you will find it to become relaxed and peaceful. Out of quietness we summon up energy from inner sources, and soon you will notice a better connection to your intuition. Your private and professional lives become more harmonious.

Some people find it easier to do the exercise with voice instructions. This is easily achieved by using a tape recorder. State the instructions very slowly, and leave enough pauses in-between to feel the different body parts.

Practising attentiveness can be very useful if you have difficulty falling asleep. You can go from the soles of your feet up your body to your head while you lie in bed. Often one does not get past the thighs.

## Outer preparation

It is beneficial to spend time making sure outer circumstances are good for treating, only starting when you have sufficient preparation and enough time. Then you can work without distraction. Disassociate yourself from the other tasks in the house or hospital. Talks and telephone calls can wait.

### The atmosphere

The surroundings play an important part and can influence what happens. Children are even more aware of the atmosphere surrounding them than adults. They react to the moods of their carers, colours, sounds and smells. A television in the background influences the general mood, flooding the senses of babies even when they are not watching it. Modern life leads to sensory overload if we do not specifically block certain things. Children cannot deal with permanent exposure to a constant stream of sounds and images. Even adults are influenced by them more than they realize. Our nervous system becomes strained, while at the same time our senses and instinct are deadened. Brutal scenes leave their mark on our souls even when we think we are immune to them. We should become a lot more selective with the things surrounding us. They colour our basic feelings and determine the atmosphere in the home.

## Warmth

The room needs to be warm. It is best if the working area is specially heated with a small heater, the pad possibly pre-warmed. Warmth is an important prerequisite. If you are cold you can neither relax nor enjoy, and babies can easily get cold.

## The place

Choose a place to massage where you are comfortable and will not be disturbed. This can be on the floor (at home), or on a changing table. It is very important to be in a comfortable position and relaxed when working, without any tension, as the hands transmit tension to the baby.

The pad should be soft. Babies almost always pass water when massaged — we should think of this and provide the necessary protection. Lay the baby on a towel or any soft cloth, in which it can be wrapped after the massage. If we want to work with oil, then keep the oil in a small bowl near at hand, pre-warmed if necessary. (Oils will be discussed in a later chapter.)

## Timing the massage

It is not always easy to find the right time to massage, as not only does the baby have to be taken into consideration, but also the surroundings: timetables and staff in hospital, other family members at home, for example, older siblings needing to go to school at specific times and still needing their parents.

There is no point in massaging if the baby is hungry or tired. The need for food has priority and has to be satisfied first. It is

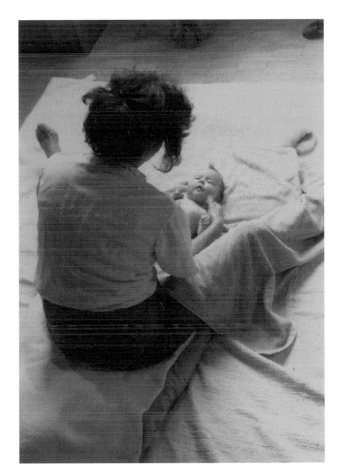

unpleasant to be woken from a deep sleep, even for a massage. It is easiest if there is a daily rhythm in which the massage has its place, as mentioned earlier. The baby gets used to it and joyfully awaits the massage. A certain regularity in daily life promotes trust in the surroundings.

## General aspects of technique and implementation

You can begin the massage when everything is prepared and you have created a place for yourself and the child. The technique is very simple, the strokes gentle and empathic, but

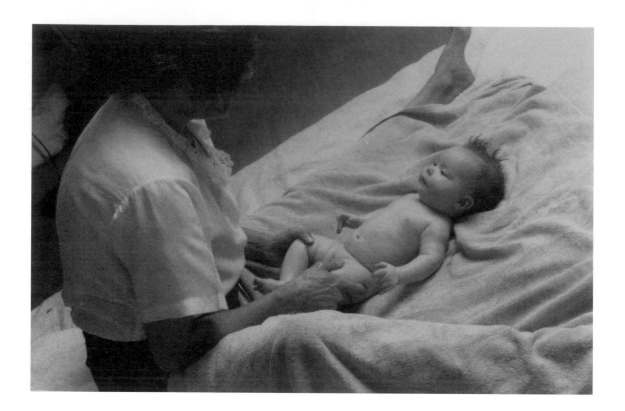

not timid. Difficult movements, complicated sequences or manipulations are not wanted, but rather loving attention.

### Getting started

The atmosphere at the beginning sets the tone for the entire treatment. It is very important that you do not feel pressed for time but work out of enjoyment. Even the way you undress the baby is part of the treatment. I usually talk to the babies and tell them what I plan to do. I take it seriously and trust that they understand me. And they do. Babies have a unerring sense for truth and sincerity. The communication does not happen through words, but in the message we convey through pitch, facial expression and body language. We cannot lie to children — they notice how

we really are and will behave accordingly.

If we do not know the child, we should leave some time before starting the massage. This is especially important if we are working in hospital, as children keep having to get used to different members of staff. As already described in the section on bonding (see page 21), it is better if babies are massaged by the same nurse as often as possible, if for some reason the mother cannot fulfil this task.

### Speaking or not?

In his book Leboyer recommends that baby massage should be done silently.[35] In my opinion this is not suitable for all children. It is good to decide each case individually. I have experienced babies who were restless and fearful if I did not talk to them. Verbal attention is important for them. As discussed, all sense organs play a part in development. We can convey affection through our voice, and I believe that babies understand the meaning of what we are saying. Humans and animals are born with the ability to understand the message of others. This understanding is not bound to words, but always comprehends the underlying truth. It is self-evident that we should not talk to or be distracted by, other people during treatment. The effect of treatment would be greatly spoiled by such behaviour.

## Trust your hands!

Do not worry about the different strokes, even if you are not used to massaging. Trust your hands. Let your hands feel: warmth, coldness, consistency of the different muscles, contours, joints. Work as much as possible with your whole hand rather than your fingertips. Your hands will nestle against the form of the body. They stroke, knead and *model*. Your whole attention is in those hands, and the more your hands observe, the more pleasant it is for the child, and the deeper the effect. The child will react to your concentration and dedication and follow your strokes and its own sensations. It will give you clear feedback and conduct a dialogue with you. You will soon find out what it likes and how different strokes affect it.

## The strokes

The strokes for different methods are described and illustrated in detail in the next chapters. The general rule is:

*The strokes should be performed*
*slowly and rhythmically*

There is a big difference in the effect depending on whether we work fast or slowly. Let yourself be massaged to test the effect. It is incredibly relaxing when somebody slowly and rhythmically strokes our body. Fast strokes stimulate and are invigorating. The atmosphere changes. Slow strokes are steady and we have a better chance of sensing what is happening in our body — and enough time to reflect on our bodily and emotional feelings.

Overall, strokes have the following effect:

*Slow strokes are calming.*
*Fast strokes are stimulating.*
*Downward strokes are calming.*
*Upward strokes tend to stimulate.*

> *While massaging let both hands stay in contact with the body — even if only one hand is working. The inactive hand holds or just lies on the body, completing the circle of energy.*

Continuous contact is especially important if the person — child or adult — is new to massage, or if they are experiencing strong emotions. Feelings of abandonment and fear can be triggered by the unexpected removal of hands. For this reason it is important to keep a bowl of oil within reach. This way you can reach the oil with one hand when necessary, while the other hand stays on the body. Using a bottle requires two hands to get at the oil, which means discontinuing contact. Handling a bottle interrupts the flow of our hands and is distracting.

## The Pressure

The pressure of our hands should always suit the weight and health of the baby. When a child is older and is used to being massaged, the pressure will automatically become stronger. Never press or manipulate. Massage is like a dance. Take your lead from the person being massaged and react accordingly. That is why attention is so important. Children will give us clear feedback and will let us know when they have had enough. They have a wide range of signals to communicate with.

Most beginners tend to be too timid because they are afraid of hurting the child. This initial reservedness will quickly pass with a bit of practice. Even fine strokes need a certain amount of decisiveness. Have faith in your abilities. It is good to avoid timidity, as your thoughts and insecurity will be observed by the child.

It appears to be a paradox, but pressure works in the following way:

*Small, fine strokes stimulate.*
*Firm strokes are calming.*
*Painful pressure blocks and causes tensing.*

## From top to bottom

In general, baby massage is done from top to bottom, unlike Swedish or sport massage. This often confuses people because they have learnt that massage should always be done moving towards the heart. With baby massage it is different: the goal is different from the one desired in sport massage. Sport massage aims to soothe pain, break down waste products and accelerate their removal, and stimulate circulation. The best way to do this is by working towards the heart. Baby massage aims to calm and relieve strain. Stroking downwards releases bottled-up energy and is calming and relaxing.

Parents and workers are often surprised how quiet they become themselves when they massage a baby, partner or friend. Massaging is not only a gift or hard work. The opposite is often true: after a successful treatment the giver also feels happy.

| |
|---|
| *Massage is a process of mutual giving and receiving* |

# IV. Action and Treatment

## Baby massage according to Dr Leboyer

We touch heaven when we lay our hand on a human body.[36]

Baby massage is the best-known method of the various methods of tactile stimulation described below. It is part of an eastern tradition and, as far as I know, also an African tradition. Supposedly baby massage was also used by Europeans in earlier times. I have encountered older people who remember how their parents or grandparents massaged babies. At the beginning of the 1980s baby massage was brought back into western consciousness by the book *Loving Hands: The Traditional Art of Baby Massage* by Dr F. Leboyer, which inspired a new generation of parents.[37] He described the type of massage he had encountered in India and documented it with beautiful photos. Since then, many books have appeared on the subject, although the massage techniques of the different authors barely differentiate from each other.

More and more parents are massaging their babies and are delighted with results. The children's development is noticeably good, and some mothers have observed above-average motor co-ordination in their children at around two or three years of age. Such experiences are passed on, and midwives, paediatric nurses and health visitors are increasingly asked for instructions. In many hospitals in Switzerland baby massage forms part of the training for nursing staff. New mothers, if they wish, are shown how to do it either in a group or individually before taking their baby home.

Baby massage is described step by step on the following pages. I would like to emphasize again that the instructions are not there to be followed rigidly at the cost of spontaneity and enjoyment. Always use your inner knowledge, feelings and intuition, and react to the signals that the baby gives you, then nothing can go wrong. The instructions are there to give initial security. Soon you will develop your own way of massaging. Babies are our best teachers.

As mentioned before, the pressure of the strokes and the length of the massage should fit the size and health of the baby. If the baby is still small you should massage gently and without pressure. The stronger the child gets, the firmer the massage should be.

For a very small, premature or severely sick baby the polarity, kangaroo or RISS methods are better suited. If you are unsure which method is the best, read the chapter on contra-indications (see page 88). You will see that there is a suitable treatment for every case.

If the baby is suffering from one of the following it is better not to apply the Leboyer massage:

— a high temperature
— acute infection
— inner bleeding
— an undiagnosed, serious illness
— swollen lymph glands

Otherwise you can massage daily. It is best to incorporate massage into your daily rhythm — the more regularly you massage the baby, the more obvious and longer lasting the benefits will be.

A full massage usually lasts about twenty minutes, although this is only a guideline. You are at liberty to massage for a shorter period of time, or to only treat part of the body. A shorter or partial massage given with intense concentration is better than a mechanical or hectic complete massage. Quality is more important than quantity. Always work with your feelings and intuition.

## The order of baby massage

| | | |
|---|---|---|
| 1. | Chest | Stroke from the breastbone over the ribs to the sides. |
| 2. | Diagonal | Stroke diagonally from the hips to the opposite shoulder and back down to the other hip. |
| 3. | Arms | With the baby on its side, starting from the neck and the shoulder, massage the arm, including the wrist, the backs of the hands, the palms and every finger. |
| 4. | Abdomen | Alternating with your left and right hand stroke downwards, circle around the abdomen beginning at the naval, and glide down the abdomen with your lower arm. |
| 5. | Legs | Same as for the arms; ankles and feet are important. |
| 6. | Back | One hand massages the back in long sweeps from top to bottom, while the other hand holds the buttocks. Then massage the muscles either side of the spine with your fingertips. Stroke across the back. Stroke down over the feet. |
| 7. | Face | From the centre to the sides. Gently knead and pull the ears. |
| 8. | Exercise | Gymnastic exercises are done to finish off. |
| 9. | Final touch | Wrap the child warmly and rock it, possibly feed, bathe or lay it down to sleep. |

Each movement is described in detail below.

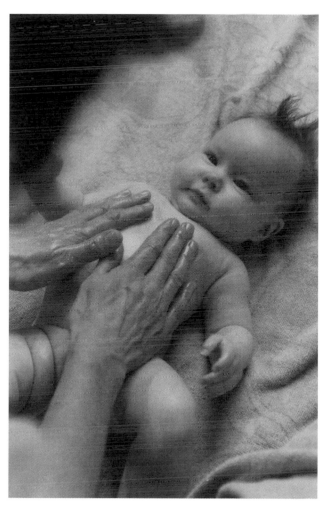 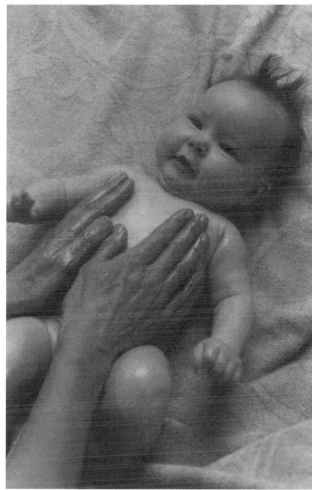

## 1. Chest

Lay your warm hands on the baby's chest and wait until it has got used to the touch. Touching the chest can cause quite a strong reaction: stretching, deep breathing, blushing. Because of this it is important to start slowly and gently. Take your time. Take two or three deep breaths and blow all the air out of your lungs. When both of you are completely at ease, you can begin the massage.

Spread some oil over the chest and shoulders to help your hands glide. Then stroke with both hands from the breast bone to the sides. Gently and rhythmically stroke in bands across the ribs and to the side of the rib cage.

Once there, do not glide over the skin back to the breast bone, but remove your hands and start stroking from the breast bone to the sides again. Stroking back and forth stimulates too much. If the child is very young or has never been massaged before, I leave one hand at the side while bringing first the one hand, then the other, back to the starting position. This guar-

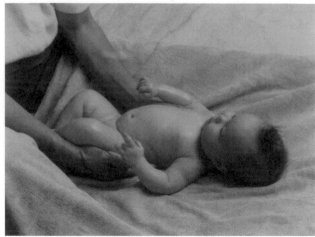

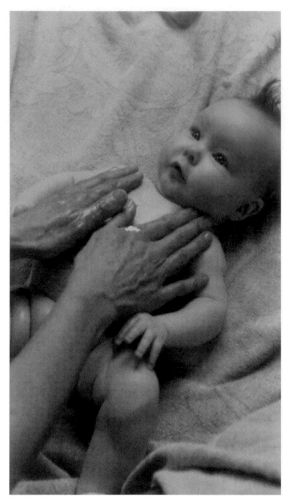

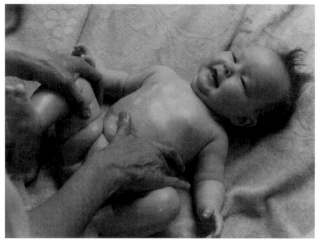

antees unbroken bodily contact, as some children get frightened and start crying if you let go of them.

I also stroke upwards and over the shoulders into the folds of the neck a few times, feeling the curve of the shoulder joint. While stroking, my hand moulds completely to the shape of the body.

Once I have stroked outwards across the chest in this way a few times, I glide along the sides to the hips. I massage the hips and the hip joints. Most babies love this!

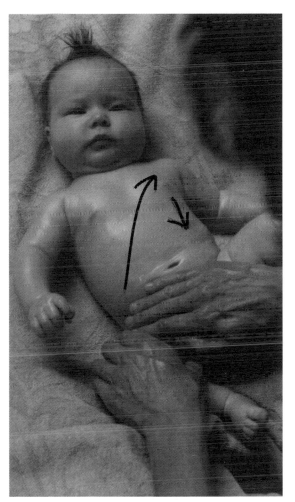

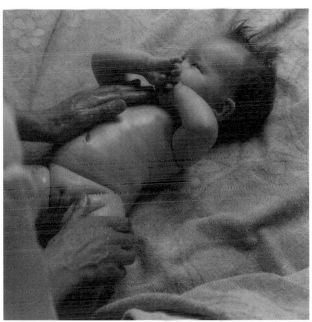

## 2. Diagonal stroking

Place your left hand on the right thigh.

Stroke diagonally upwards with the right hand from the right groin to the left shoulder, and glide down the left-hand side to the hip joint.

To reverse, hold onto the child's left thigh with your right hand, and with the left hand stroke diagonally upwards from the left groin over the abdomen and chest to the right shoulder, then down to the right hip joint.

Repeat these strokes about three times.

(Course participants are sometimes confused by this diagonal move. But do not worry, it sounds more difficult than it is.)

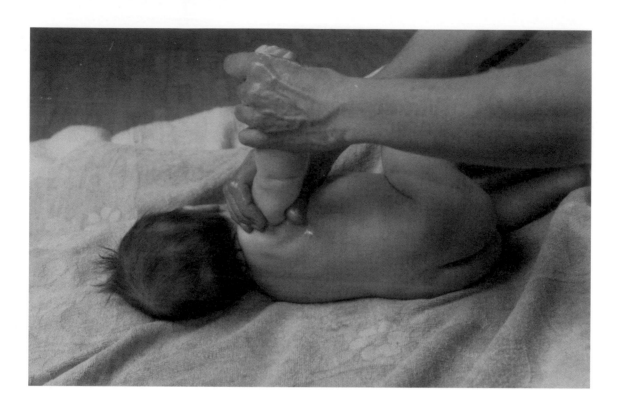

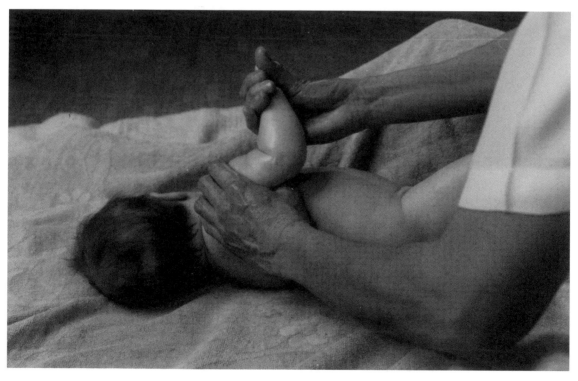

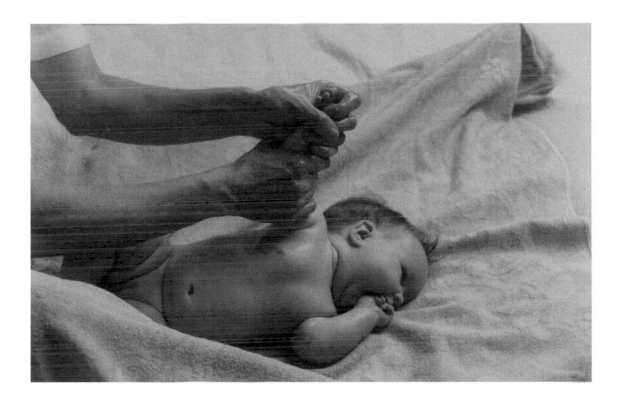

### 3. The arms

To massage the arms, lay the child on its side so that the shoulders and neck are easily reachable. Do not force it, if the baby objects, leave it lying on its back.

Spread more oil over the arm.

Use your 'inner' hand to hold the wrist, while the other one massages the neck and shoulder. Work from the neck over the shoulder to the shoulder joint and loosen the muscles and joint.

Usually the arm will relax, and you can pull the arm by the wrist and straighten it a bit, so that you can reach around and knead the upper arm. Twist your hand around the upper arm with a kind of 'milking' movement, pressing and releasing the muscles.

Continue in this fashion down to the lower arm. Once at the wrist, change your grip. The 'outer' hand should now hold baby's wrist, while the 'inner' hand starts massaging the upper arm down to the wrist.

Massage the arm in this way two or three times, making sure not to forget the elbow.

It is also good to stroke once or twice up the arm from the wrist to the shoulder to get rid of waste materials.

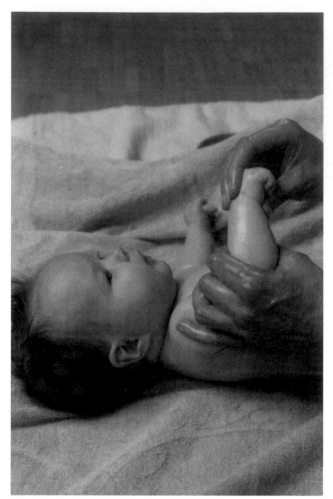
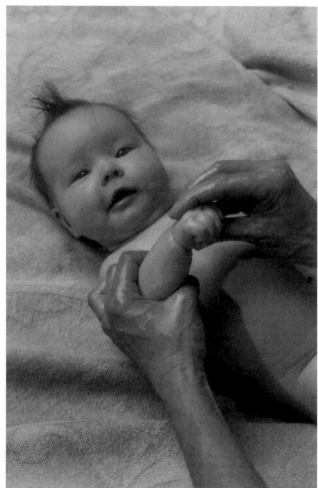

*Hands and wrists*

Joints are important transitional points where energy often bottles up. Loosen the wrist and massage around the wrist with your fingertips and thumb.

Massage the 'padding' on the back of the hands — most babies love this.

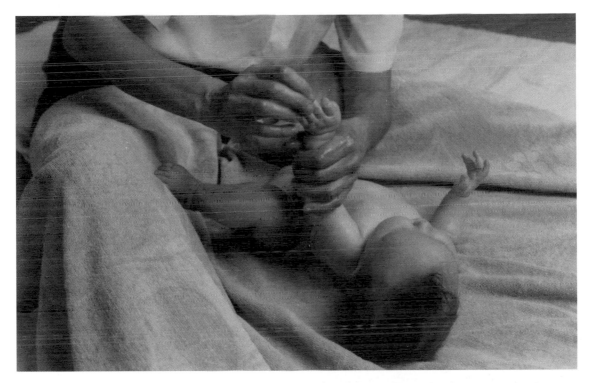

Every finger, from the little finger (pinkie) to thumb, is stroked around and then stroked upwards. Usually the hands loosen and can be opened easily for massaging the palm. Never force a child to open its hand.

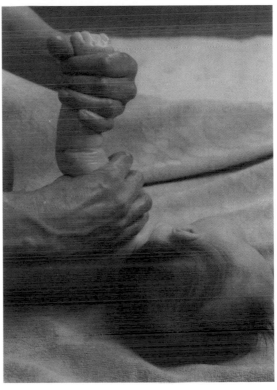

Finish the arm massage by 'wringing out' the arm: clasp around the arm with both hands and rotate them in opposite directions from the upper arm to the wrist.

Then turn the baby onto its other side and massage the other arm in the same way.

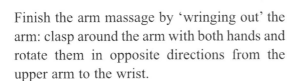

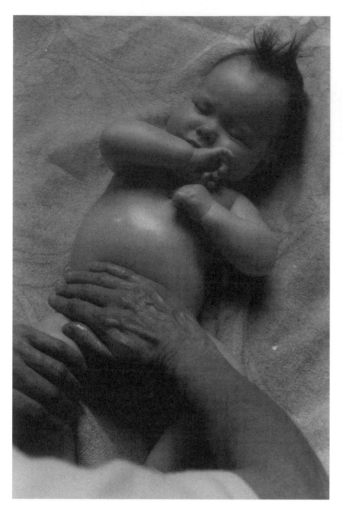

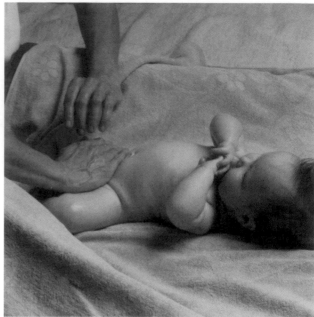

First rub the abdomen with oil.

While doing this it will become clear whether the area is soft or tense, empty or full. Some abdomens are very soft and yielding under the hand, so that it is possible to apply good pressure. Others are hard and tense. In that case, pressure is not suitable, and it takes time — possibly repeated massaging — until the tension is released. Notice whether the stomach is full or empty. After a full meal it is better not to massage.

### Centre of abdomen

Glide across the abdomen with alternate hands from the pit of the stomach to the pubic bone, with as much pressure as the abdomen allows.

## 4. The abdomen

The abdomen is the area below the ribs.

I have often noticed in courses that learners of abdominal massage often reach up into the chest area. This stimulates the heart and can be too stimulating. We have already massaged the chest area at the beginning. Now we should stay in the soft areas of the stomach and gut.

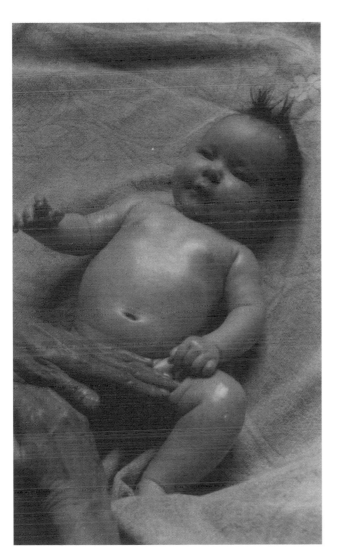

If you feel that the abdomen is hard, try and relax it first. Rocking can help. Slip one hand under the back and support the small of the back, with the other hand hold onto the abdomen and gently move it back and forth, or gently shake it. If you have relaxed it through gentle shaking and vibrating you can continue with the abdominal massage. When you gently press into the abdomen in the following strokes, the abdominal wall should be soft and yielding. A child who is very tense may need several treatments before it relaxes.

Glide downwards with the whole flat of your hand, tilting slowly up to the edge of the hand.

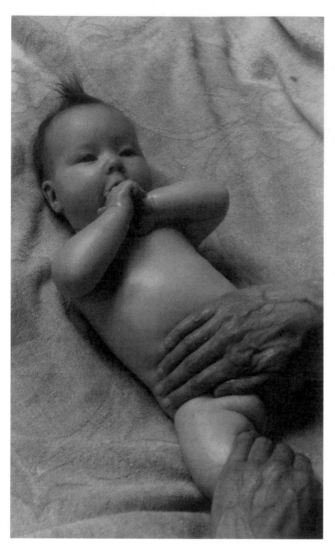 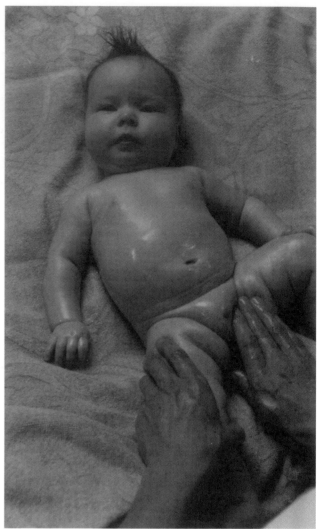

*Stroking the abdomen, sides and groin*

With your right hand stroke down the right side from the base of the ribs over the groin to between the legs and over the genitals. Neither make a big fuss about the genitals, nor leave them out as if they do not exist or are untouchable.

Repeat the same movement with the left hand on the left side of the abdomen. Repeat this move a few times, alternating between the left and right sides.

Boys can get an erection when their abdomen and groin are massaged. This is a normal reaction and can occur even in tiny baby boys when they are relaxed, warm and content.

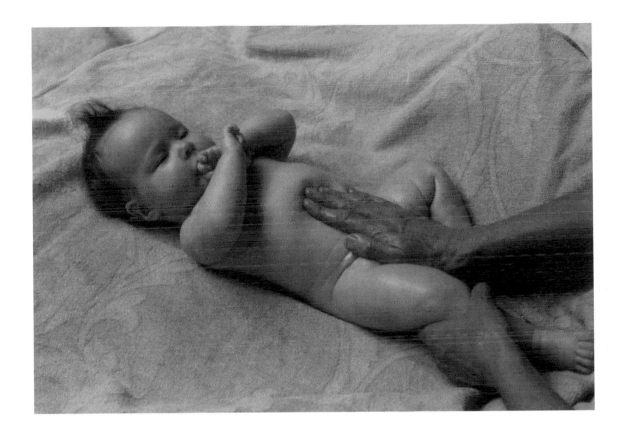

For many centuries it has been drummed into us that there are 'indecent' areas of our body. In this regard we are very uptight. It is known that we shape the later attitude of our children to their body and sexuality through our behaviour — and especially through our repressed and unconscious feelings. Eventually we may realize that we are not as uninhibited as we think. Because of this we should observe our own reactions to such situations. The feelings that emerge when sensuality plays a part show us what our basic, and possibly unconscious, attitude is.

## Circling on the abdomen

Start circling the naval with the fingertips of the three middle fingers. Circle around the naval first, then spiral outwards with a little pressure. Let your fingertips be very observant. The abdomen can tell us a lot about the condition of the baby.

**Important;** These circles should always be *clockwise*, so that we are supporting the movement (peristalsis) of the colon; that is, in the same direction as food is transported through the colon.

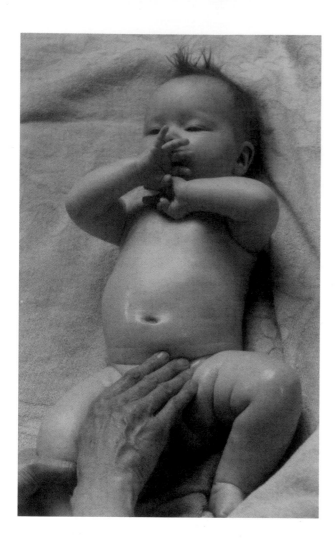

Many children love abdominal massage so much that they stretch out towards our hands and make all sorts of happy noises. However it is also possible that a child is reminded of painful colic and cries (see page 40, "the inner attitude").

*Stroking downwards with the lower arm*

For this movement hold the legs upright with one hand — to relax the abdominal wall — and stroke down the abdomen to the pubic bone with the whole lower arm. Do this two or three times. Many children also enjoy this!

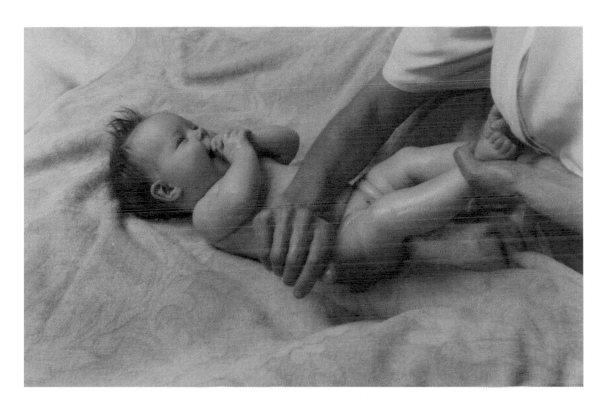

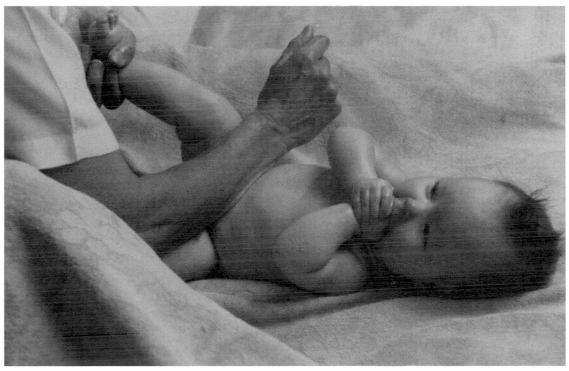

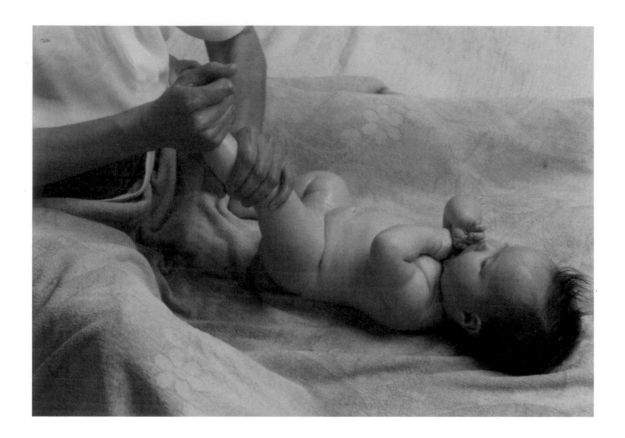

## 5. The legs

For the legs follow the same principles as for the arms (see page 57).

One hand holds the ankle and keeps the leg upright, the other hand massages rotating and 'milking' from the thigh to the ankle.

As with the arms, firmly stroke from the ankle upwards once or twice to help get rid of waste material. Stroking downwards relieves tension. Both are helpful.

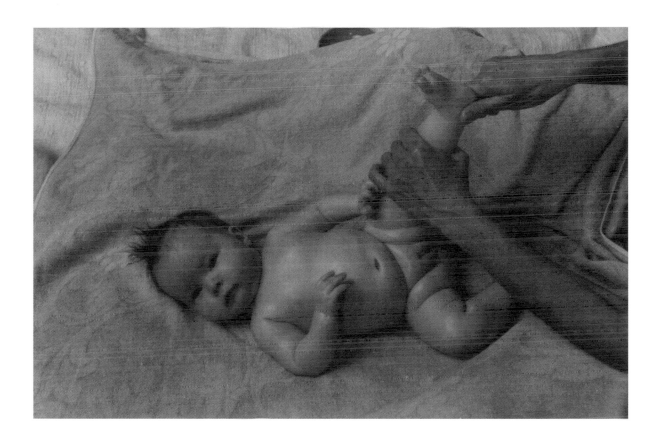

### The Foot

Stroke repeatedly down the foot joint with your hand moulded closely to the contours. This 'connects' the leg and foot.

For the foot massage, hold the leg up by the calf with one hand while the other hand massages.

Work around the ankle, your thumb massaging on the one side, your fingertips on the other.

### The Instep

Circle around the fat pads of the instep with your three middle fingertips.

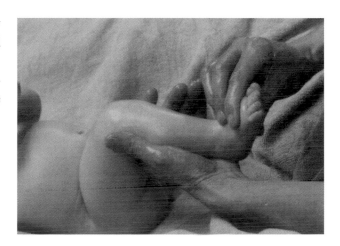

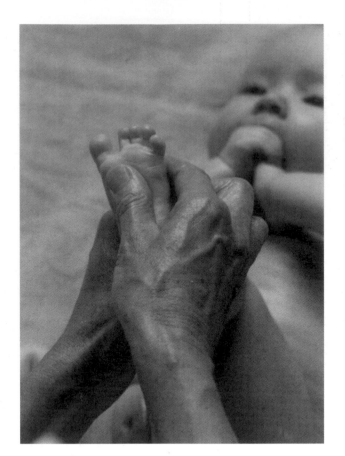 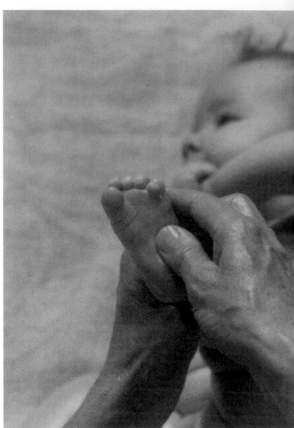

*The Sole of the Foot*

Stroke with your thumb across and circle clockwise over the whole sole. Your touch can be quite strong. Remember that too gentle a touch can irritate or tickle. Circling the sole clockwise can help to relieve constipation.

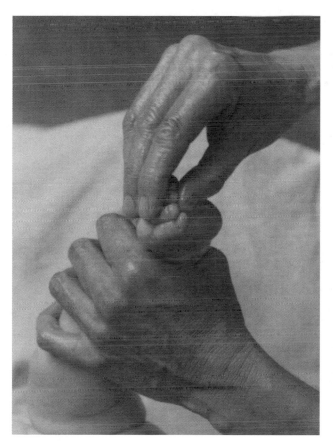

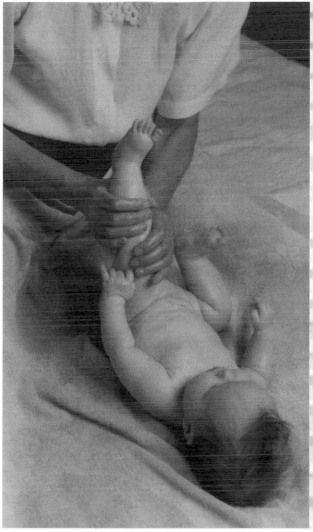

## The Toes

Start with the smallest toe, with your thumb on the underside, and the index finger and/or middle finger massaging the upper side. Pay attention to everything, feel every little joint, every curve.

## Finishing the leg massage

Finish the same as for the arm by kneading the whole leg again from thigh to ankle. 'Milk' by circling both hands in opposite directions (as for the arms).

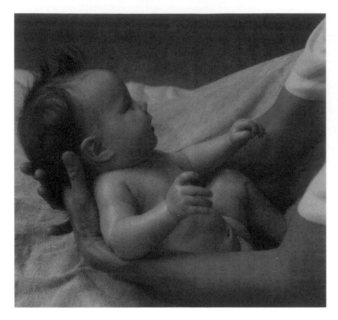

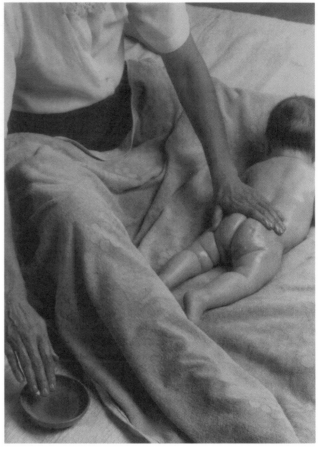

When you have massaged both legs, turn the baby onto its stomach and lay it down sideways in front of you ready for the back massage. It is easier to stroke and hold in this position.

Have a quick chat before turning the baby around.

## 6. The back

First spread oil over the back.

### Stroking downwards

Hold the buttocks with one hand to keep the baby steady and stroke down from the neck to the buttocks with the other hand using long, rhythmic strokes. Treat the whole back in this way with long, downward strokes, and massage in sections from one side of the back to the other. Let your hand mould snugly to the contours of the back. Do not

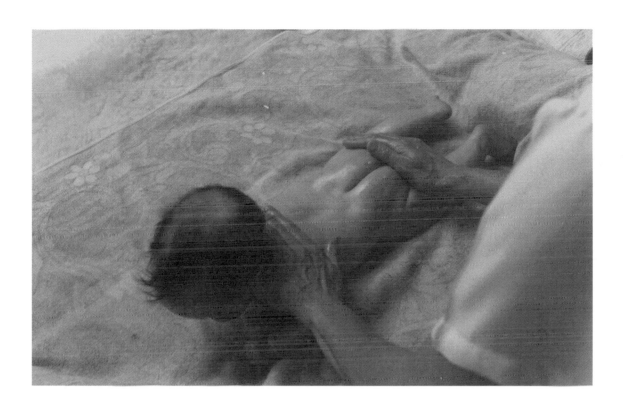

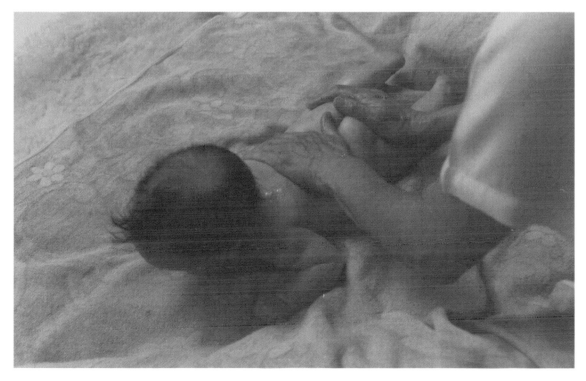

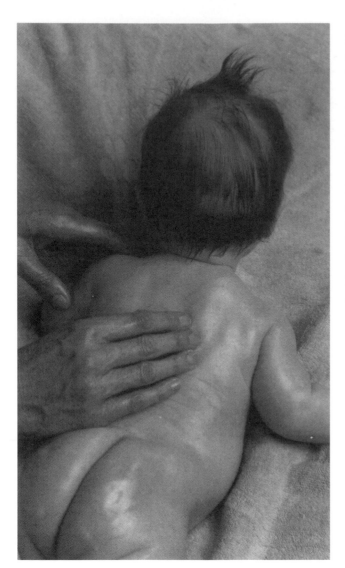

forget that the more attentively you observe everything, the more effective the treatment will be.

*Loosening the muscles*

After a few long, downward strokes the back muscles can be treated in more detail.

Do not use the whole hand for this, but the fingertips of the middle three fingers. Circle and loosen the muscles along either side of the spine, down to the dimples in the small of the back. Remember to keep both hands on the body, even when only one of them is working. Lay the passive hand on the shoulder, for example.

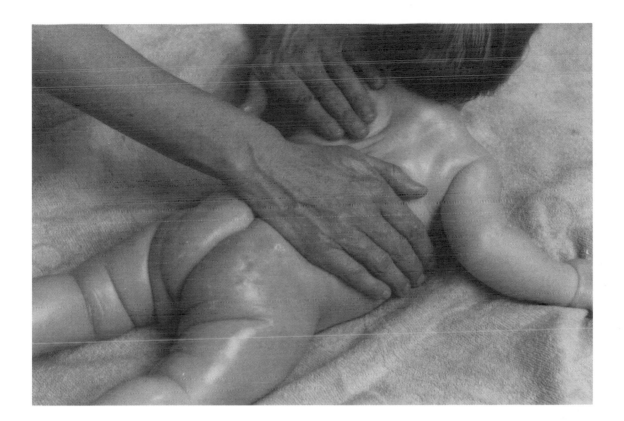

*Side stroking*

Stroke back and forth with your hands perpen-
dicular to the spine, each hand moving in the
opposite direction to the other. It is all right if
the skin is moved around a bit.

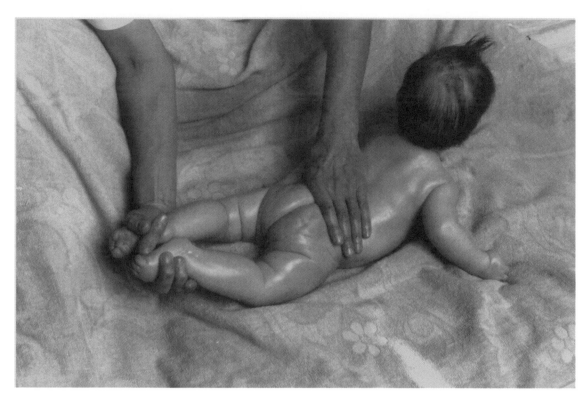

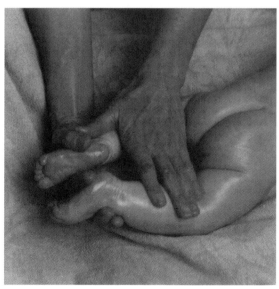

*Finishing the back massage*

To finish, stroke two to three times down the whole back with sweeping strokes. Starting at the forehead, stroke back over the head and shoulders and down over the feet and beyond. It may be helpful to imagine that loosened tensions are being wiped away. Then turn the child onto its back again to start the face massage.

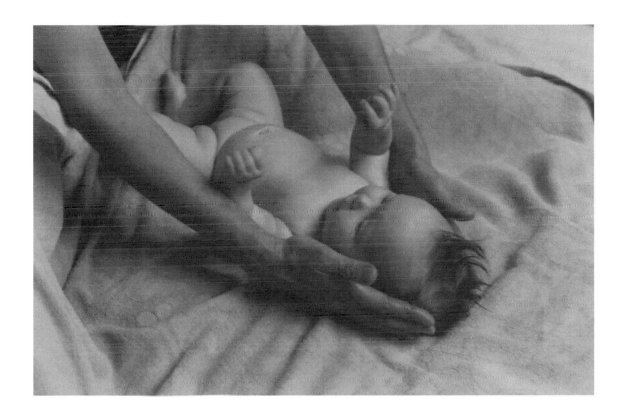

## 7. The face

Not all children like to be touched on their face. Do not force it!

Stroke with both hands over the forehead, across the top of the head and down the sides to behind the ears.

Then stroke with both thumbs from the middle of the forehead to the sides. Begin at the hairline, and work your way down in bands to the eyebrows, always starting from the middle of the brow. Only stroke from the middle to the sides (do not apply pressure to the temples), then lift your hands and begin again in the middle.

As mentioned for the chest massage, if the baby is very scared or small, bring the thumbs one after the other to the middle, so that the body contact remains unbroken.

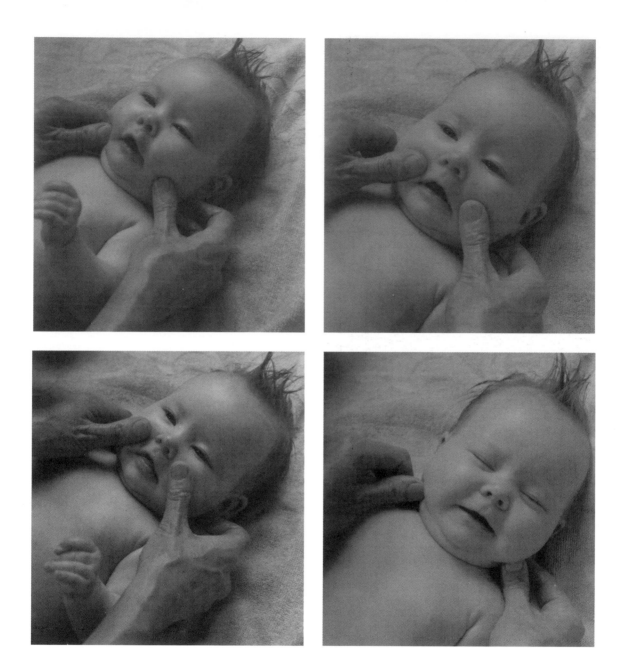

Stroke from the bridge of the nose over the nose and cheeks with the thumb or fingertips. Do not worry about the exact path the movement takes, the bone structure will lead you.

*Upper and lower lip*
Here again, stroke from the middle to the sides in bands until you arrive at the chin. Stroke from there to the ears.

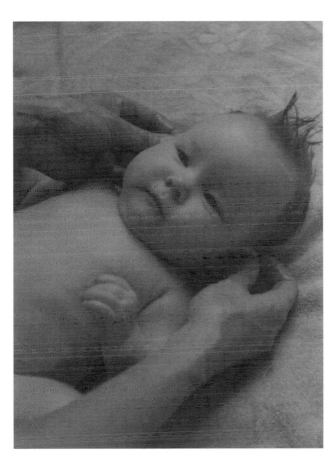

## The Ears

I massage the ears by grasping them with thumb and index finger, lightly kneading them and then gently pulling. Try it out on your own ears — it feels good!

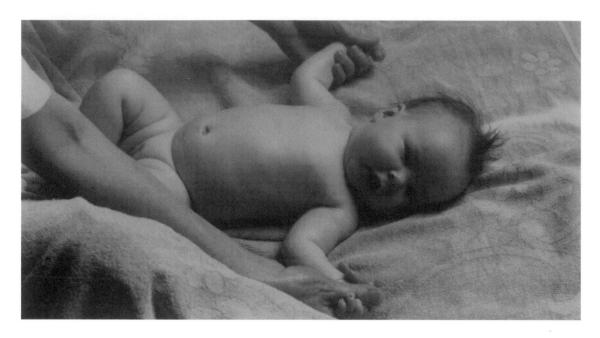

## 8. Exercise

Leboyer recommends ending the massage with a few gymnastic exercises. Repeat every exercise two or three times.

### Both arms

Open out both arms wide (they are usually very relaxed after the massage) and then cross them over the upper body.

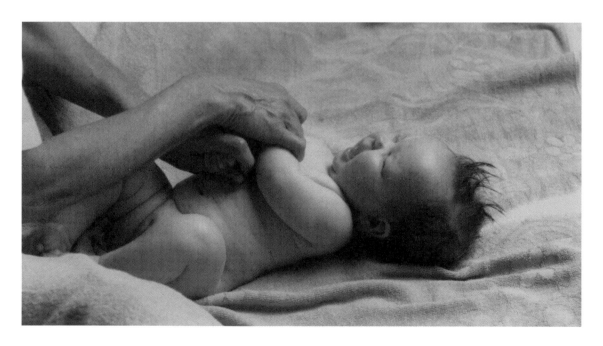

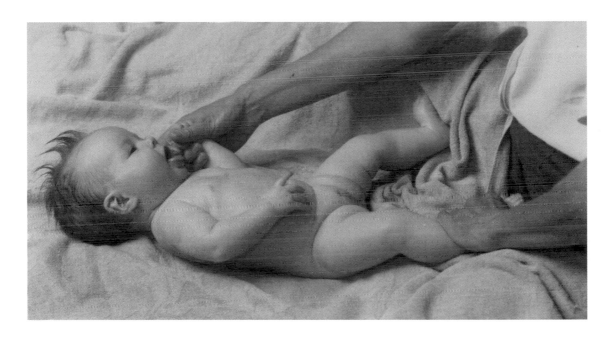

## One arm, one leg

Next is a diagonal movement: one leg and the opposite arm are stretched out diagonally and then pulled towards the middle of the body.

This movement makes many children giggle.

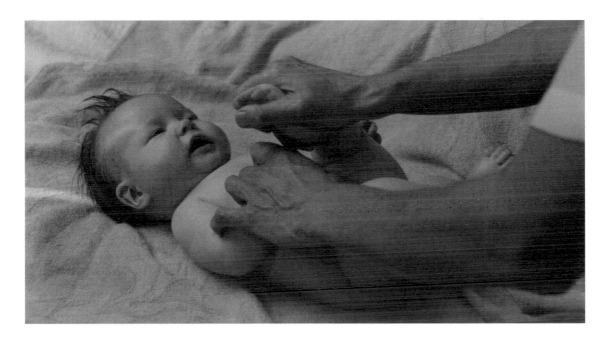

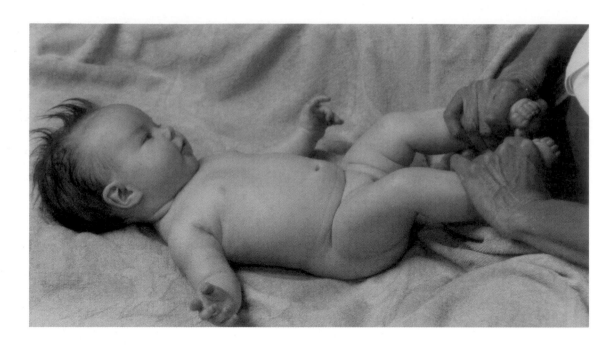

### Both legs

The legs are brought up and crossed over above the abdomen. This has a good stretching effect on the small of the back and the back.

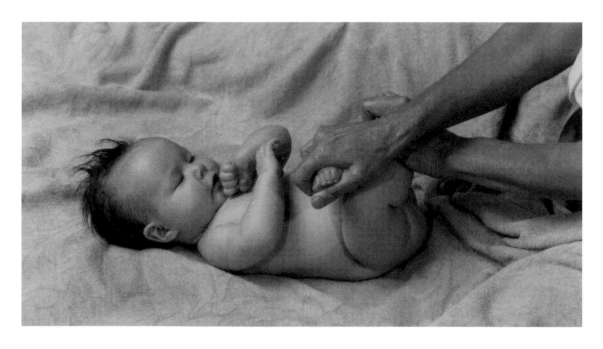

## 9. The final touch

The treatment is now finished. The baby can be wrapped in a cloth and rocked. Leboyer recommends a bath after the massage, but possibly the child will prefer to sleep as such a treatment can be very tiring, or it may be hungry and needs to be fed.

Do not be surprised if it sleeps deeply and for a long time afterwards.

### Do not forget

Remember that for different reasons it is not always possible to give the whole massage. Do not be disheartened by this, but remain flexible. You can start with a short back or foot massage. This does not mean you are doing less. Whatever is enjoyable is also healing, and a partial massage will have an effect on the whole body. Even 'only' a small foot massage will be good for the whole person. With time, the treatment will automatically become longer.

### A few tips for learning

It might initially appear difficult to follow the instructions out of a book. But with a bit of imagination it can work well. I have learnt to imagine in my head what I have read — first the single moves, then the whole process. I shut my eyes and imagine the child (or adult) and in my imagination give it a massage. Our brain treats this visualization in the same way as a real massage. Once we start treating for real we have already practised and it will be easy to start.

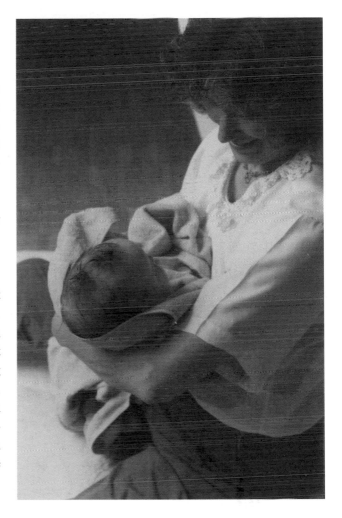

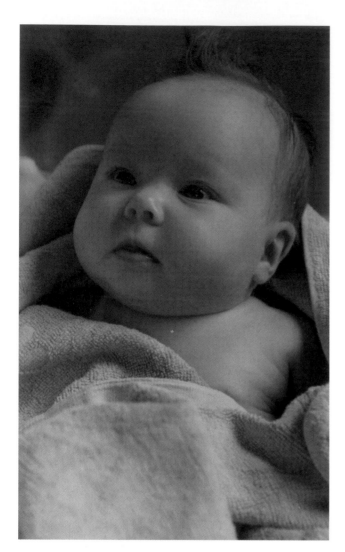

We learn best if we treat ourselves to a massage now and again! With every massage we receive we learn more and become more sure about giving. Courses in massage help to deepen and strengthen your knowledge and ability. Courses are not only useful to practise techniques, but also give the opportunity for self-development and self-experience. We also develop a more conscious and more loving relationship to our own body and can reduce our fear of touch. It is also important to experience with our own body what we wish to transmit or recommend to others. This is especially true if you are in a job where you want to teach massage, for example, as a health visitor, nurse, midwife or therapist or in the maternity ward.

> *It is important to experience with our own body,*
> *what we want to apply and impart to others.*

I wish you lots of enjoyment!

# Different oils

Oil is used for baby massage (although it is not essential for the RISS method). It helps our hands to glide smoothly over the skin without creating unpleasant or painful friction. There arc many available oils, but not all arc suitable. It is important that they come from an organic source; products, including lotions, that contain mineral oil arc not suitable.

> We should use only high quality vegetable oils and, if possible, only cold-pressed oils.

Mass-produced, commercially advertised massage oils can contain non-organic oils made from non-edible petroleum. Always check the ingredients of all products before you purchase them. If you cannot find out about the ingredients it is better to avoid the product, however nice it smells. Even the term 'baby oil' is no guarantee of quality or organic oils.

Stick to simple, natural vegetable oils which agree with the skin and are absorbed well. Then you can be sure there are no artificial perfumes or other additives.

## Disadvantages of non-organic oils

Mineral oils are dead matter and the skin does not absorb them well. They do not contain any nutritional value, do not support the functions of the skin and possibly interfere negatively with the uptake of vitamins. Adele Davis notes that:

Vitamins A, D, E and K have a tendency to dissolve in the mineral oils that are often used on small babies. The oils sink through the skin into the blood connecting to these vitamins, which are then flushed out of the body in the stools. This causes vitamin deficiency.[38]

## Keeping vegetable oils

Vegetable oils should be kept in dark, airtight bottles. After some time they turn rancid and become unusable. Because of this it is sensible to buy small quantities. Jojoba oil keeps for longer than some other types of oil.

## Simple vegetable oils

As already mentioned, different, if possible, organically produced, vegetable oils are suitable for massage. Cold-pressed oils are qualitatively better and contain more unsaturated fats. It is perfectly acceptable to use cold-pressed sunflower, olive or almond oil.* They can be used on their own or as a base oil for mixing or infusions with herbs and flowers. Of these, almond oil is the most popular. It is mild, inexpensive and easily available.

## Oils from healing plants

Knowledge about the healing properties of plants is widespread in Switzerland. In nearly every household you can find several herbs that can be used in teas or baths to cure various ailments. They can also be used for

* Almond oil should be avoided if there is a history of nut allergy in the family.

massage. Such oils are available in chemists or can be made at home by infusing the plant in the oil for several weeks.[39] I would like to stress that plant oils are not the same as essential oils, which are discussed in the next section. Plant oils are much milder. The following oils are suitable for regular massage or for treating a specific ailment.

### Melissa oil (Melissa officinalis L.)

Melissa is good for flatulence, and is calming and uplifting. A mild nerve sedative, it promotes sleep and strengthens the heart.

### St John's Wort oil (Hypericum perforatum L.)

St John's Wort flowers in the summer and has a strong connection to the sun and light. It gives energy. I know of an anthroposophical clinic where they massage children who have circulatory problems with St John's Wort oil. It also strengthens nerves and heals wounds, as well as helping skin function through hypericin which helps the skin absorb more light. A midwife told me she uses this oil for newborns with jaundice. The baby is rubbed with the oil and then laid in a sunny window with as few clothes as possible, although still kept warm. Never use St John's Wort as a sunscreen, you can be burnt even when there is only a bit of sun.

### Camomile oil (Matricaria Chamomilla L.)

Camomile loosens cramps, helps pain relief, stops infections and heals wounds. This wonderful plant, also accepted by allopathic medicine, is an old remedy and eases intestinal problems such as; colic and flatulence, as well as soothing itchy skin. Camomile can occasionally cause an allergic reaction, so try it out first on a small patch of skin.

### Avocado oil

Avocado oil contains valuable minerals and vitamins (especially vitamin A), which are absorbed by the skin.

### Rose oil (Oleum rosae L.)

Most people love the smell of roses. Roses affect our feelings, making us joyful and calm and help us to sleep. Rose oil is also a disinfectant. It is very good for skincare. It should be diluted with avocado oil or almond oil — 5 drops of real rose oil to 100 g of base oil.

**Important:** when buying rose oil you have to ask for *real* rose oil (which is very expensive). Otherwise you will automatically be given an artificial product sold as rose oil.

## Essential oils

Please distinguish between plant oils and essential oils. As mentioned above, essential oils are not the same as a healing plant infusion in a carrier oil. Essential oils are the *essence* of the plant and thus have strong healing properties. They should not be used routinely, but only consciously and specifically for ailments. In his book *Aromatherapy*, Tisserand advises against using essential oils for babies and small children.[40] This is understandable, as these oils contain the essence of the plant in its highest concentration. Not only chemical compounds, but also plant substances can be harmful in high doses and inappropriately used!

Essential oils have more applications for adults and older children: in massage oils, baths and oil lamps. Some examples were described in the chapter on birth (see page 16). The aromas work through respiration and the sense of smell. They are absorbed through the skin and exhaled via the lungs. Essential oils should not be used regularly or thoughtlessly in high concentrations. They have so much strength that one drop of certain plants can have a strong effect, although rose is the least poisonous. Essential oils are useful for older children and adults to treat problems like sleeping disorders, restlessness, fatigue, tension etc. Their scent brings joy into the house and purifies the atmosphere.

As with other oils, it is also important where you buy your essential oils. You should aim for the best organic quality. Artificial scents are not suitable for healing purposes. To test for authenticity, put a small drop of the oil onto a piece of paper. Unlike other oils, real essential oils do not leave any marks on the paper.

# Simple, supplementary steps

*The healing property of water*

The element of water is suitable for supplementing or finishing a massage. Water is one of our oldest healing elements. It relaxes, invigorates and cleans — not only dirt, but also flushes electrical tension out of our system. Water strengthens the immune system. Gravity is overcome to a large extent in water, which relieves our organism. Most newborns feel good in water, as it is the element out of which they have just been born. Leboyer recommends a bath at the end of the massage, so that it flushes out any remaining tension.

The Russian researcher, Tjarkowsky, has had great successes with his water cures with sick children and babies. He discovered the method when doctors had given up hope for his very ill daughter. He decided to take the baby home against medical advice and try saving her himself. He laid her in water, for hours at a time, and the baby grew and flourished. He discovered that the amount of energy needed for bodily functions was dramatically reduced in a condition of lessened gravity. He wrote:

> A further effect of water which promotes the growth of the foetus is that the organism needs 60–70% less oxygen in a state of weightlessness. A much smaller part of the available oxygen is needed for upholding bodily functions.[41]

Most of us know the pleasant effects of a bath. It is worth testing how a baby feels in water and holding it for longer periods in a warm bath, if it has a calming influence. Even a small foot bath can show surprising results.[42]

*The skin — an important organ for detoxing*

Our skin provides an important contribution in the detoxification of the body. Often we can smell the condition of an ill person by their body odour. Mothers can tell if their babies are experiencing teething troubles, or if they are about to go down with 'something' by changes in their babies' smell. Mrs Breindl, the famous expert on Hildegard-medicine, told me that every childhood illness has a specific smell which can help diagnose the illness. She learned this from the famous Professor Sauerbruch, with whom she worked as a young nurse. He was supposedly able to tell by the facial expression and smell of a baby whether its parents were alcoholics or not. He apparently asked his teams: "Can't you smell it? It's so obvious."

The detoxification of the body via the skin plays an important role in our health. Since our organism is now much more burdened by things such as environmental pollution or unnatural foods with artificial additives, our skin needs special attention. The skin should be well supplied with blood and have the right pH-value so that it is able to fulfil its important detoxification function.

Modern bath products should not be used. Babies do not need perfumes, especially not artificial ones. Pure baby skin does not need shower gels nor lots of soap. These things obstruct the skin functions rather than having a use, and can attack the pH balance of the skin. The difficulty for parents nowadays is not trying to provide essentials for the baby, but choosing the right things and protecting their children from the surplus of industrially produced, completely unnecessary products. The simpler we remain, the better. Leaving out is almost always the best option, however convincing the advertising campaigns.

One simple method of supporting the detoxifying function of the skin is to maintain the acidity barrier by adding a few drops of vinegar to laundry or to bathing water, especially for babies with mothers who are heavy smokers or drug addicts, or who are on heavy medication.

> *Put one tablespoon of vinegar into a baby's bath or load of laundry to maintain the acidity barrier of the skinand to support detoxification.*

Perspiration and the skin's ability to breathe are blocked by disposable nappies and clothing made from artificial fibres. If a baby remains in a wet nappy for too long, its skin will reabsorb the poisons secreted with great effort by the kidneys. It is important that particularly sick babies and those undergoing drug withdrawal are changed regularly, and cleaned with water. Wet wipes, although convenient, often contain alcohol which is unsuitable for the skin and can be reabsorbed.

> *Disposable nappies and clothing made from man-made fibres impede the function of the skin.*

The following chapter discusses methods for treating sick and premature babies.

# V. Gentle Tactile Stimulation for Sick and Very Small Babies

## Too early, too small, too sick

Premature and sick babies need particular care and attention, although they are often especially isolated, and there is still concern about how much 'handling' such babies can cope with.

Maternity wards in Switzerland have changed completely in the past ten to fifteen years, inspired by figures like Leboyer and Odent. Parents are well informed and know what they want. Mothers whose babies are born on time expect to be able to care for them themselves, and to have their babies with them at all times. However, the situation is less clear for mothers with premature or sick children. Many ask themselves what they can do, or what they are not allowed to do. The high-tech atmosphere in intensive care is unfamiliar and frightening. Most of us need some encouragement from doctors or nurses before we feel free to move around in such an environment. Some hospitals realise the importance of the mother-child relationship especially for premature babies. A video from the Academic Centre in Amsterdam illustrates this well.[43]

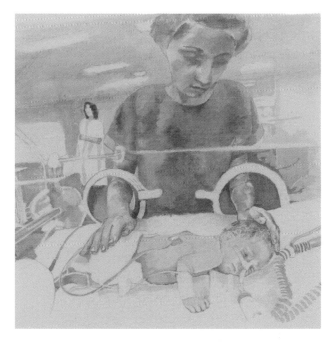

The women's clinic in Bern has been using baby massages and the kangaroo method successfully since 1989, and also offers complementary treatments. Mothers can choose from many remedies, for example, reflexology, Bach flowers or meridian therapy.[44]

I would like to encourage parents whose baby is in intensive care to look after their baby as much as possible themselves, even if the setting is unfamiliar. Ask to be involved in and informed of, all aspects concerning your child. Ask to be shown how to care for, wash and feed it. The following pages will show you examples of how you can give your child a lot of bodily contact. Have faith in your feelings: the longing to touch, carry and stroke. Do not be put off these interactions by the unfamiliar surroundings of the intensive care ward. You are giving your child the best chance to thrive.

Before describing different techniques for premature and sick babies I would like to include some thoughts on contra-indications to dispel any fears or doubts. Where touch is concerned, we appear to have quite irrational fears and resistance, but it is a great shame to withhold a loving touch for fear of doing damage. Take some time over this question to increase you confidence when treating.

# Contra-indications for treatment

## *Healthy children*

There are no contra-indications for healthy children for the body treatments described in this book. However, it is better not to give a massage if the baby has a full stomach, or would rather sleep. Never force a child or yourself if neither of you are in the mood for giving or receiving a treatment.

## *Premature and sick children*

It is not easy to answer the question whether to treat a very small or sick baby. I have not come across much information on this subject. Probably nobody has dared to set up guidelines in the knowledge that there can be no one definite procedure.

You will need to judge each case individually, and continually reassess your decision for every crisis situation. It is not easy to assess how much 'handling' a high-risk baby can cope with. Because of this these babies often receive fewer loving touches for fear of harming them.

This does not have to be the case. However critical the situation, a baby should never have to do without loving and healing touch, as we can always help in some way. There are different techniques — the more critical the condition, the gentler and finer the treatment has to be. After consulting the doctor and nurses, and depending on the condition of the child, you can choose a suitable method. This could be the kangaroo method or RISS method, or laying your hands on the baby (polarity) if the baby cannot be moved. Only when the baby's health has stabilized should you use baby massage.

## Polarity (see page 93)

Polarity is the gentlest of all the techniques. You can *always* use this wonderful way of giving energy and attention to sick people, by laying your hands onto their body — even with the tiniest babies, and with severely ill or dying people, regardless of age.

## The RISS method (Rice Infant Sensorimotor Stimulation Technique)

The RISS method is also called 'loving touch'. It can be performed either by parents or staff.

Dr Ruth Rice developed this method specifically for premature and newborn babies. She also treats sick babies, and has had impressive results. While in a hospital in New York, I experienced how she treated a tiny boy who weighed no more than a kilogramme. The RISS method is suitable for premature and weak, sick children, as you stroke very gently. I personally asked Dr Rice about any contra-indications. She did not know of any, but could remember one premature baby, whose skin was so delicate — like tissue paper — that she preferred to keep her hands above the skin and work with energy fields.

This treatment is also suitable for babies in incubators. You do not need to use oil for the RISS method, which makes treatment easier. Unlike the Leboyer and other usual baby massage methods you do not 'knead' or 'milk,' but work with gentle strokes. This

means you can use this treatment even when you do not want to subject the infant to a firmer massage.

The RISS method was tested in the USA according to scientific principles. The differences at all levels of development between the treated children and the control group were so striking that this method has now been employed by many large hospitals in Europe and America. The research results have found international renown.

## The Kangaroo method (see page 102)

You need to decide individually whether a baby is ready for the kangaroo method — in critical periods from one hour to the next. The decision to start the kangaroo sitting is dependant on many factors and will rely on the doctor's verdict.[45]

## Massage (see page 51)

There are a few restrictions with the baby massage of Leboyer and others. Length and intensity of the treatment have to be tailored to the circumstances, as we have already described in detail. As this method works deep into the tissues, there are some situations when it is better not to massage (see page 52 on baby massage).

With high-risk babies you need to assess whether the skin is functioning well, especially with babies of heavy smokers or drug addicts. It is a sign of good skin function if the baby urinates when it is stroked. Feel the glands, if the lymphatic glands are swollen you should not massage.

Concerning contra-indications, it could be said that in the industrial countries we have harmed our children in the last two to three generations by *not* touching them. Already one generation back parents and nurses were not allowed to stroke and cuddle newborn babies in hospitals. Babies were taken away from mothers as soon as they had finished breast feeding and taken to the sterile, inaccessible maternity ward. The main reason for this was the emphasis placed on hygiene, in order to avoid illnesses and complications. Also the idea prevailed that babies should be left alone. But hospitals that allowed mothers into the intensive care units reported definite advantages. There was no increase in infectious diseases and studies showed that parents took more heed of the hygiene rules than staff.

## Sensorimotor stimulation with high-risk babies

*Do we touch very ill babies too infrequently because we are afraid of harming them?*

This is a very important question, because insecurity and fear can stop us from giving a sick baby much-needed bodily contact. This subject was discussed by specialists in a conference for 'sensorimotor stimulation of high-risk infants.'[46] The issue of whether tactile stimulation could cause negative physiological reactions like apnoea* or bradycardia† in high-risk newborns was discussed in depth.

Here is the answer that Dr Gluck gave to this question:

We developed the first intensive care

---

*   *Apnoea*: a temporary cessation of breathing
†   *Bradycardia*: a condition in which the heartbeat is slower than normal (less than 50 to 60 beats per minute).

unit for any term and premature infants in 1960 at Yale ... The biggest problem we faced was how do you give care. Bill Silverman, who was my own mentor, used to teach that insofar as possible one must never disturb the baby. One must leave them alone. We have gone from there to doing all sorts of things to babies, but without knowing how much handling is essential or how much is detrimental. That was a real problem then, and so it continues today ...

I subscribe fully to your thoughts about handling the baby right from the start and particularly the ill ones who ordinarily never get any attention except procedures. Infants in incubators are even worse off because they are subject to about 90 decibels of continuous noise, and bright lights shine 24 hours a day in their faces. We all agree this is a very unhealthy atmosphere. Nevertheless, there are some aspects of technology that we must cope with, and that precludes many of the stimulating procedures that one would like to try. Another important aspect, of course, to remember is that if one opens the incubator and holds the baby, the infant becomes cold, and, as we know, this is detrimental. Unfortunately, the fact is that neonatal stimulation has not been carefully worked out. Although we feel strongly positive about some of these stroking techniques, we actually don't know how much stroking is enough, and how much may be too much. Some of us even have tried to emulate with the premature the weightless atmosphere that the baby had in utero, such as with water mattresses. However, at this time, we are not clear on just how this ought to be done and on its value. Overall, one of the things that I suspect will become blazingly bright and clear during this conference is that although we have made great strides in salvaging babies, we may have gone 14 steps backwards in how we actually give care to them. Our care actually may be inhumane.

About 1961 we started to bring mothers into the Special Care Nursery. At that time this was against the law. I regret we never actually published that we were doing this, but since it was against the law, we never said much. At that time we became convinced that there was no question bu that the parents made a tremendous difference in recovery of babies. To us this has always seemed clear, that no matter how sick a baby is, the mother ought to be putting her hand on the baby and handling the infant. To me there is no question about the necessity for handling but I hope information about how much and what kind of handling will come out of this meeting.

As we can see, even an experienced paediatrician like Dr Gluck had no general procedures for when and how a child should be treated with one of the tactile methods, but he is convinced that sick newborns need bodily contact and should be stroked. And he thinks it a matter of time before we find out how much, and what kind of, 'handling' is right for a child. I do not believe that it is right to have fixed, general rules about contra-indications. There never will be a generally valid treatment, because we are talking about humans with their own feelings and completely different responses to stress. Every child is unique and deserves an individual decision and a personal treatment; flexibility, empathy and intuition are necessary characteristics in a carer. I know that intuition is not officially asked for in scientific areas. Medical science is concerned with measurable values of the physical world and likes to depend on concrete laboratory results; it demands measurable and repeatable results, valid for any situation. How ever, we live in a period of renewed thoughts concerning these views. Modern physics states that there is no such thing as an objective experiment, as not only thoughts and attitude, but also the mere presence of an observer can influence results. If we are honest we have to re-evaluate the previous seemingly *secure* basis of science, leaving a bit more room for the heart.

Dr Rice spoke in the above mentioned conference about her experiences with tactile stimulation in severely sick premature babies. She felt that the tactile and kinaesthetic stimulation should be started immediately after birth. Kattwinkel indicated that tactile stimulation reduces the incidence of apnoea in premature infants.[47]

Then she spoke of an experience that she had at a seminar in a hospital in Tennessee. She walked into the nursery for premature babies, and all the nurses wanted to see a demonstration of the treatment. She felt that she had to make an impact, because this was the first time they would see the treatment being used. She looked for the smallest and sickest infant in the nursery, and chose a 900-gramme baby who was 46 hours old and was in an incubator. He had not yet opened his eyes, or moved. She began to stroke him and in about 10 minutes he gained some colour. The nurses noticed that he was getting pink. Then he urinated.

Although Dr Rice didn't know the significance of the urination, she knew that this had been observed in other babies. Susan Ludington used a modified version of Dr Rice's stroking technique with the babies she had studied. She found that infants who were stroked urinated significantly more frequently than those weren't, and in greater amounts. The little infant at this hospital in Tennessee yawned, opened his eyes, and began to move around. Dr Rice felt that as a result of the stimulation, he became alive. Her conclusion was that sick infants should not be deprived of touch.

## Gentle massage for premature infants

From *The Harvard Medical School Mental Health Letter*, September 1987:

> What is the worth of infant massage? We asked Tiffany Field, PhD, Professor of Paediatrics and Psychology at the Center for child development at the University of Miami Medical School, Director of the Debbie School nurseries ...
>
> Infants who are born prematurely or endure a difficult birth are more likely to have learning disabilities, suffer child abuse and develop mental health problems. In a recent study of children aged four to ten years who had been treated in a neonatal intensive care nursery, 49% were found to suffer from depression, conduct disorders, and other psychiatric problems. One possible contributor to this, in addition to organic impairment associated with prematurity, is the disturbance in early interactions between these infants and their parents. The cause of the disturbance is not entirely clear, but it is possible that parents become overprotective because they regard the baby as fragile ...
>
> Adults find massage calming, and the same might be expected of newborn children. Parents are apparently aware of this, since they naturally stroke and massage babies ...
>
> Supplemental stimulation makes babies stronger, less fragile-looking, and more responsive; as a result, parents interact with them more sensitively. Massage is one of the most effective forms of stimulation, partly because physical contact allows quick detection of over-stimulation. If a baby tenses its muscles and squirms, the parent is able to modify the amount or intensity of stimulation immediately, without having to wait for signs like fussing or crying.
>
> Premature babies treated with massage in the neonatal intensive care nurseries show superior growth and development. In one study we provided this treatment to 20 infants born at an average weight of less than three pounds after an average of seven months gestation. They were given 45 minutes a day of gentle massage (15 minutes three times a day) for ten days. First the infant was laid on its stomach and for five minutes the therapist provided tactile stimulation, gently stroking the baby's head, shoulders, back, arms and legs with the palms of the hands in a set pattern. Then the infant was turned over on its back and for five minutes the therapist provided kinaesthetic stimulation, gently moving its arms and then its legs. Finally the

infant was turned over again and the tactile massage was repeated.

After ten days infants given this treatment had gained 47% more weight than a control group. They were also more alert and active and scored better on a standard test of newborn beahior, the Brazelton Neonatal Behavior Assessment. They were discharged from the hospital an average of six days earlier (a saving of $3000 per infant) and were healthier and more responsive when the parents assumed care of them. Eight months later their interactions with their parents were less disturbed and they performed better on tests of development.

We do not know yet whether they will have fewer mental health problems than the infants who did not receive massage, but it seems likely that the better relationship with their parents will result in better relationships with other children, and they will be mentally healthier or at least happier.

I would like to end this chapter on contra-indications with this report. I hope that spreading such clear evidence inspires specialists and parents. Loving touch and stroking is not a new medical discovery, but a most natural reaction. Disturbances that develop through neglect and lack of touch are immense, we know that now. Evidence has shown without doubt that tactile treatments not only help in coping with the stress of intensive medical care and to reduce complications, but also that they further the child's whole development and the parent-child relationship.

# Specific treatments

## *Polarity*

The polarity method is possibly the oldest art of healing — laying hands onto the body. Holding and placing hands on another person is an instinctive gesture, used to give attention and sympathy and to reduce pain. As mentioned in the section on contra-indications, the laying on of hands is always an appropriate treatment, regardless of how serious the condition. You need not worry about treating a tiny or severely sick child with polarity. It is amazing what energy and effectiveness lie in these simple gestures. The child becomes more peaceful and relaxed when it feels our hands. Pain and separation become more bearable. Loving touch and protection lessen stress and reduce complications. Polarity is especially appropriate for critical phases, sick babies or babies in incubators. It is beautiful to see how the facial expression changes during a treatment and becomes tranquil and content. I also use this method for terminally ill adults, and notice how patients become very peaceful. Typically reactions are: relaxation, deeper breathing and general ease. One very ill, old lady beamed: "now it is quite light in my body." Often patients fall asleep. But even if we do not notice any outer changes in very sick patients, whether newborns or the very old, our efforts are not in vain. Attention of this kind is never a waste of time and is good even if there is no obvious feedback.

There are no restrictions regarding length or frequency of the treatment in polarity. You can use the technique as often, and for as long, as you want. The more the child experiences loving, calming hands the better. You can also practice it after meals and during sleep.

The polarity method is also appropriate for busy members of staff in intensive and paediatric care units, who want to give their patients more attention and positive experiences. The treatment can be done over clothing and thus does not need much preparation. You can use any chance to lay your hands on a patient to create a short moment of peacefulness. For parents this method is a welcome opportunity to become active and help their baby on their visits to hospital. The polarity method differs from a spontaneous laying on of hands owing to the specific body positions that it works with, and which are suitable for receiving and distributing energy. These are the so-called poles, from whence our touch works most effectively from an energetic point of view. The technique is incredibly simple. You do not need extended training or a degree. Your empathy and your wish to help are your qualifications.

## Method

I would like to remind you of the basic rules described in Part III (page 39). They are true for any kind of treatment — and thus also for the polarity method.

Concentrate completely on the child and do not be distracted by other happenings in the room. The treatment cannot be good if we talk to other people at the same time. This is a bad, but widespread, practice — talking over the heads of patients. Even if a baby does not react it still needs our full attention.

It is best to tune in before the treatment and centre ourselves. This means coming to ourselves and becoming completely peaceful inside by breathing deeply in and out a few times. Then observe the baby intently, watch its breathing, its expression, feel in what state of mind it is. Then you can begin treating. Place your hands slowly and carefully onto the body, leaving them in the same place for several minutes. Always work with both hands. They should lie with practically no pressure or should be held one or two centimetres above the body. The effect is still there even when there is no physical contact. This variation is suitable if certain areas are painful, for example, with burns, over a plastercast following hip operations, or if too many instruments obstruct the body, and so on.

We actually transmit energy with our hands. There is an energy point in the centre of our hands, whose colours and light can be photographed with modern technology. In old paintings of the saints, you can often see these shining energy centres with their rays of light formed on a blessing gesture. Our hands can also 'bless.' They transmit vibrations, as our voice expresses emotions. What our hands radiate and mediate depends on our thoughts and feelings. Because of this I have already stressed the importance of attitude during treatment. Here I would like to repeat that ambition and the expectation of specific results arise from our ego. This undermines our serenity and calm and disturbs the process. One should never try and manipulate life energy.

For the polarity method let your hands rest for one or two minutes on the chosen body parts. When you remove your hands, let them rest a few centimetres above the treated area for a moment before removing them completely and going on to another area, or ending the treatment.

These are a few of the polarity movements you can choose from:

Rest your hands without pressure on the body, or one or two centimetres above the body.

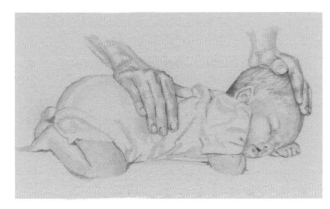

*Abdominal position:*

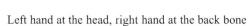
Left hand at the head, right hand at the back bone

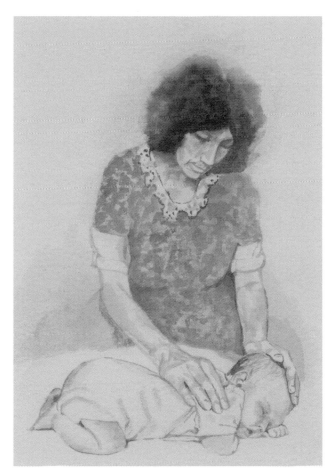

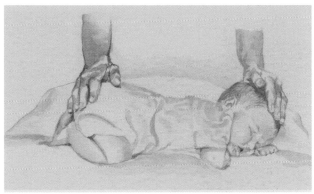
Left hand at the head, right hand on the backside

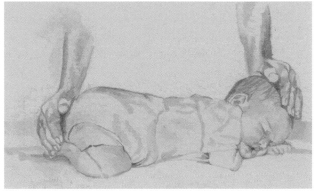

Left hand at the head, right hand at the chest area

Left hand at the head, right hand on the soles of the feet

*Back position:*

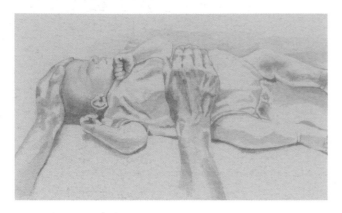

Left hand at the head, right hand on the abdomen

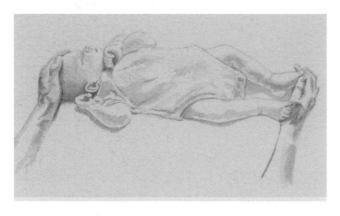

Left hand at the head, right hand on the soles of the feet

It is worthwhile repeating these moves throughout the day.[48]

## The kangaroo method

Babies react so positively to the kangaroo method that many hospitals have started using it. Evidence has shown that premature babies develop better and their chance of survival significantly increases.[49] Parents who have been encouraged to use the kangaroo method with their premature babies are delighted with the results. It is obvious that their babies are doing better. They themselves are also incredibly relieved because they do not have to watch passively and can develop a rewarding intimate relationship with their child.

Even more so than with full-term babies, it is important that parents are actively included in the developmental and healing processes of premature and sick babies. The kangaroo method is suitable for this, and we should not withhold this simple and effective treatment from anyone. I encourage parents to use this method as often as possible when they visit their child. Instead of sitting next to the bed or incubator, let the baby lie on your chest. Tell your paediatrician and nurses what you want, and ask them to assist you with the kangaroo method.[50]

### Method

Let the mother or father sit on a comfortable chair with an adjustable back rest. (A rocking chair is particularly suitable). The mother sits comfortably, and adopts the position which is the most suited to the present condition of the child — upright or leaning back. Then her baby, wearing only a nappy, is placed on her naked breast and covered with warm cloths. The baby lies in warmth and security and has

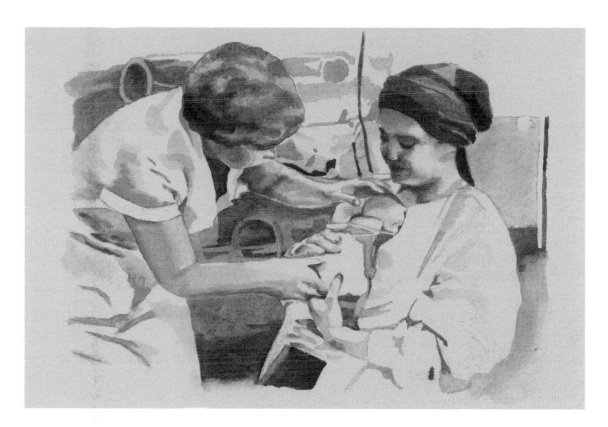

A nurse helps with the Kangaroo method

a restful break from all the strong sensory impressions of the incubator and the painful medical interventions it is usually subjected to. Here it experiences a completely different, loving nourishing touch. Even babies who show sensitive reactions to other nursing duties relax during a kangaroo sitting and show stable vital statistics. The sittings can be hours long and can be repeated during the day. Using the kangaroo method both babies and mothers flourish!

Whether a premature baby is ready for the kangaroo treatment depends on various factors and each case should be individually considered. The paediatrician will evaluate the condition of the child and will decide, from a medical point of view, whether the treatment can be started. As Ludington described, she even works with babies who are attached to breathing machines if the general condition allows. In the chapter 'Is my Child Ready for the Kangaroo Method?' she writes:

Whether a child is ready for a kangaroo sitting depends on many factors. The birth weight alone is not sufficient. I saw a tiny baby with a birth weight of 800 grams who was ready for its first kangaroo sitting after two weeks because a newly-developed surfactant treatment led to early improved breathing facili-

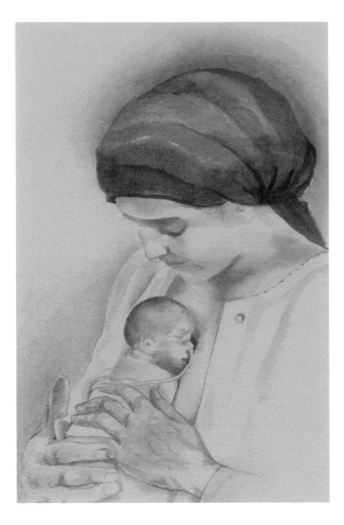

— The baby is in an incubator or an open bed.
— The medication is constant.[51]

Dr Ruth Rice describes a programme which was implemented by Dr Edgar Rey and Dr Hector Martinez in Bogota, Columbia with support from UNICEF, and which received worldwide interest.[52]

In the San Juan de Dio hospital 11,000 babies are born each year and care for those that are premature was poor because of the shortage of staff, medicine and equipment. In 1979, in a desperate and creative attempt to ensure the survival of more of these prematurely born infants, Drs. Rey and Martinez introduced a procedure that the native mothers had used for centuries. They called this alternative approach 'the kangaroo method.'

They asked UNICEF to support a study to take place in the San Juan de Dio Hospital. They named it the Home Care Low Birth Weight Programme. Using the kangaroo method, survival figures for very low birth weight babies (500–1000 grammes) in the programme rose from 0% to 72%. For those who were born at a weight of between 1000 and 1500 grammes, the survival rate rose from 27% to 80%. The programme was also successful in enhancing mother-infant bonding, which in turn promised consistent good care from the mothers.

UNICEF made the information from the study available, and in the 1980s many hospitals in Sweden, Norway and Finland began to use the kangaroo method in their Neonatal Intensive Care Units with infants who required assisted ventilation.

Staff and parents were delighted with the

ties. On the other hand I have seen a 2500 gramme birth weight baby whose treatment required so many tubes and continuous nursing it prevented any kangaroo treatment.

In general we give a green light for treatment in babies over 1500 grams, if the following criteria are fulfilled:

— The pregnancy was at least 28 weeks long or the conception age is at least 30 weeks (the pregnancy plus the following weeks of life).
— The breathing device is stable.

infants' rapid improvement. Many changed from artificial to independent breathing. Apnoea was greatly reduced. The first controlled study was conducted in Düsseldorf and showed good results. In 1989 Rice introduced the kangaroo method to the Mautner Markofschen hospital in Vienna. Parents and nursing staff were delighted with the babies' physical and psychological reactions to the close bodily contact with their mothers. The children were allowed to remain with their mother as long as they wanted. That could be 1–3 hours a day.

The physiological and psychological advantages of an upright position and skin to skin contact with the naked breast and nipples of the mother could be a strong impulse for growth and development.

You can expect the following results from the kangaroo method:

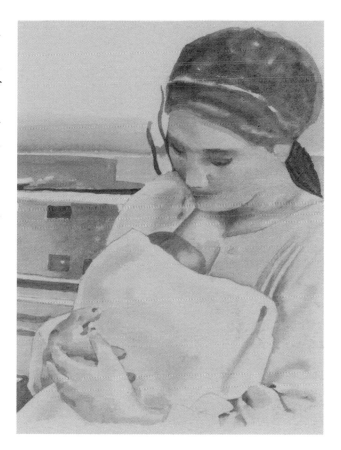

'Nesting' on mother's breast

1. Less irregular breathing and less apnoea.
2. Faster weight increase.
3. Babies are warmer on their mother's breast and retain a constant body temperature. Often mothers and babies appear to be in thermal synchronicity. The temperature of the mother rises when that of the baby falls.
4. Oxygen pressure (TcP02) remains more constant, which excludes certain complications.
5. Practically no crying during 'kangaroo.'
6. The infant is calmer and more attentive and enters into more eye contact.
7. A slightly faster heart beat, which is a positive sign, as bradycardia can be a problem.
8. There is no increase of infection with these children.
9. The possibility to breastfeed increases as the babies lie close to the nipple. Mothers tend towards breast-feeding for longer and produce more milk than other mothers breast-feeding their children.
10. The babies have a characteristic expression of joy and calm on their face, which could mean that the limbic system, and thus also the

immune system, is involved.

11. Babies smile earlier and more.
12. There is more opportunity for bonding with both parents, as both father and mother can practice the kangaroo method. Placing the baby onto the naked chest of a parent improves irregular breathing, which is so typical of newborns.[53]

The advantages described above seem convincing. They follow the continuum principle and fulfil a whole row of the infant's basic needs: closeness to the mother, tactile (touch), aural (heart beat, voice), and visual excitement (eye contact) etc. As studies have shown, the position of the baby's body carried on the breast supports breathing.

When reading the above publications, one can hope that this simple, extremely effective and, at the same time cost-effective method soon becomes part of any therapy for sick and premature newborns. All those involved profit from it, from the hospitals saving large amounts of money to the children.

# Drug-dependent newborns

Remember your own power, and that every time wants its own answers.[54]

I would like to mention this group of very disadvantaged children in particular, because they especially benefit from the treatment methods described here. For years newspapers have published articles about the drastic increase of babies born with addictions. For example in *Weltwoche* in 1992 Barbara Lukesch wrote:

Experts have estimated that 1500 to 2000 children live in Switzerland whose parents or mother are drug addicts. In 1987 the women's clinic of Zurich University recorded a marked increase in the so-called 'drug babies': The number of mothers who took heroin, methadone and, less often, cocaine during pregnancy increased from one to two cases a year, to 12 and now 20.

High pitched screaming, rapid breathing, shaking, sweating and cramping — these are the symptoms of newborns born of drug addicts [...] A study done by Hans Ulrich Bucher brought it to light: 31 of 425 (more than 7% or 1 in 14) showed signs of drugs in their first stools (meconium) namely opiates, amphetamines, methadone, cocaine, cannabis and sedatives.[55]

Soer and Stratenwerth write:

> Those concerned have long been aware of what German drug policies and rehabilitation have barely seen as a theme: heroin addicts also have children, and most of them try and live together with them.
>
> ... There are about 120,000 heroin addicts in Germany ... About a quarter of them have children, often more than one according to international estimations. Even with such vague guesses one can deduct that there could realistically be 20,000–30,000 children of heroin-addicted parents in Germany.[56]

Even if these estimations are too high, we still need to accept that an increasing number of children are starting life severely disadvantaged because of their mothers' alcohol or drug dependency. Some of them suffer severe withdrawal symptoms. According to Soer and Stratenwerth there are no official numbers for babies born with addictions in Germany, and they mention that sometimes withdrawal symptoms are not even recognized in some hospitals. One can hardly imagine a worse start than to be born with an addiction. Being alone with pain and fear is incredibly stressful and uses up the energy necessary for survival. The tactile methods described here are particularly suitable for these children: polarity treatment or massage are very beneficial and can be repeated several times a day for 5–15 minutes. Carrying these babies, and the kangaroo method seem intuitively correct in these cases.

For children of drug addicts Bach flower remedies can also be very helpful (see page 111). They can lessen panic and stress, and can be given simultaneously with other drugs without risk. And — an important plus in a hospital routine — Bach flower treatments do not take up any time. In the following section on Bach flower remedies some suitable blends are suggested.

It is worthwhile trying baths because the infant can possibly relax and recuperate briefly in the water element.

The earlier we start with intensive support, the better the chances to help in the first phase of life. With a large disorder like addiction regular, daily treatment is even more important than normal. The birth of a child can often be a turning point for an addicted mother. She can suddenly see a point to her life, and the new task is a strong motivation to go on with withdrawal. Women suffering from severe withdrawal symptoms are often insecure about their mothering abilities. They are helped with concrete, practical advice on how they can transmit pleasant feelings to the baby through touch, e.g. massage. It has been shown that women with damaged natural instincts who regularly massaged their babies gained more trust and a deeper relationship with their babies through these positive interactions. The ability to improve disturbed mother-child relationships is an additional, valuable aspect of massage.

The extra work — both in time and for people — involved in treating babies with withdrawal systems is immense. Daily extras such as massages and kangaroo sittings are unrealistic within the hospital routine. Staff just do not have that much time. It remains to be seen

> *Any method which serves to calm or give pleasant experiences with touch, however briefly, is invaluable.*

whether extended family members or helpers can be actively involved if the parents of the child are not able to completely fulfil this task. One could also think about using volunteers. This possibility has been successfully employed in hospitals which use 'doulas' (companions during childbirth and confinement) or 'nursing attendants,' These are often mothers whose children have grown up and who offer their maternal skills and experience. For example they *adopt* premature or sick children when their parents, for whatever reasons, are only partially, or not at all, able to take part. They visit the child at least once a day for a long period of time to give it lots of attentions and bodily contact. I experienced such a scenario in the premature unit of a large hospital in New York. A woman was standing cradling and talking to a child in the middle of all the bustle. It was explained to me that this woman had taken over the role of 'nursing attendant' and spent several hours a day with the baby.

> Children who are not able to be close to their mother often develop depression, lack of appetite, weight loss and often even a lack of energy that can lead to death. Because this has often been noticed, some hospitals are now recruiting volunteers to hold, stroke and cradle these children. (It has been said that the results are surprising).[57]

Montagu goes on to describe how an American doctor introduced this 'mothering' into his hospital:

It was Fritz Talbot who brought the idea of 'gentle love and care' back from Germany, which he had visited after the first world war, not using these words but the practice. When he visited the hospital in Düsseldorf Dr Arthur Schlossman showed him around the wards and theatre. The rooms were kept clean and tidy, but Dr Talbot saw to his surprise a large lady carrying a small, ailing child on her hips. "Who is that?" asked Dr Talbot. "Oh, that is old Anna. If we have tried all medical possibilities and the child is still not flourishing, then we give it to her. She has never failed."[58]

"Oh, that is old Anna, she has never failed." A simple, almost "primitive" method. "Primitive" according to a dictionary means original, native. *Prim* means the first, undivisable, that which comes first. Basic needs are 'primitive' and need a primitive response: large Anna, the original mother. The tubes, injections and monitors enable biological survival. The loving hands of a nurse and the warmth of a large Anna answer to a primary need no less important for survival. If we are able to combine these primary things with high-tech machines, then we can expect surprising success.

## Mothers withdrawing from drug addictions

A mother who has decided to withdraw from drugs needs all the support she can get. A withdrawal which is not viewed from a holistic perspective does not have a good prognosis. Beside the medical help she needs help on all personal levels, financial as well as social support. Every healing process depends on many factors. Substitution drugs alone are not sufficient for getting clean. While medical help, and with it psychotherapy, are offered, diet is often neglected. However, diet is one of the most important factors of holistic therapy and also plays a pivotal role in withdrawal therapy.

Addicts suffer from loss of appetite and usually have a catastrophically bad diet. Apart from that the chronic stress leads to the over use of important vitamins and minerals, which enhances malnutrition. The lack of vital nutritional substances also affects emotional behaviour; the sufferers lack energy, enthusiasm and motivation, and experience one failure after another. Nowadays we know that mineral and vitamin deficiency can change the basic character and life feelings of a person, but it is very difficult for a healthy adult to change their eating habits. For addicts who have forgotten how to pay attention to, or even notice, their bodily needs this task is gigantic. They need help with their diet: not junk food, snacks, soft drinks and loads of sugar, but healthy foods.

Even if their diet is improved, substances from food are insufficient to solve the deficiencies. Further support is needed to give the body much-needed nutrients. Orthomolecular medicine, the knowledge about the effect of nutrients, can be a valuable tool.

## Orthomolecular medicine

Orthomolecular medicine — medicine of nutrients — describes the effects of vital substances for treating different illnesses, including addiction. Dr L. Burgerstein wrote a comprehensive book on this subject:[59]

Libby and Stone: Drug addiction is a severe illness, a severe metabolic disturbance. The main reason that programs fighting drug addiction fail is because of the concept of 'criminality and punishment.' A drug addict should be treated in the same way as someone with metabolic disturbances. Every attempt to solve the problem without restoring total health will fail.

With increasing quality and quantity of drugs the addict will lose more and more of their appetite. Their diet will become worse: vitamin and protein deficiencies occur. The drug addict will suffer Hypoascorbemia-Kwashiorkor [severe protein and vitamin deficiency]. All humans lack the ability to produce vitamin C by themselves and thus the ability to produce the increased required amount due to severe stress.

A goat of *ca.* 70 kg experiencing only a little stress will produce about 20 g of vitamin C to cover its physiological needs; with physiological or psychological stress it needs 3–5 times as much.

The drug addict under immense stress will suffer physical damages if s/he does not receive additional vitamin C. The human requirement is estimated to be 20–30 gr., but the drug addict is under increasing vitamin C need, which can be fatal if not addressed. The authors describe how they rescue severe drug addicts from their addiction. The addict receives vitamin C, multivitamin and mineral supplements as well as pre-digested proteins, as their digestive system does not function properly. The doses of vitamin C depend on the level of poisoning of the specific drug, but at least 25 g are given, in some cases 3–5 times more, in single cases even more. These doses are given for 4 to 6 days.[60]

Another author, nutritional therapist B. Mäder writes about vitamin C:

Prof. Linus Pauling estimates the daily allowance as 75 mg to 12 g. Vitamin C is the general vitamin for our body, which it uses in great amounts when available. It is responsible for activating the entire immune system. It protects our body by supporting the synthesis of interferon (which works against viruses). Vitamin C is able to neutralize pollution and many chemical food ingredients, e.g. nitrate, nicotine, drugs, tablets etc. It strengthens the protection against allergies.[61]

The amount of vitamin C needed varies greatly and depends on many factors such as infection, stress etc. With modern pollution and dietary habits including unnatural, unripe food the daily required amount of vitamin C cannot be met. Infectious diseases lead to a great increase in the amount needed. Because of this the amounts suggested by the different authors vary greatly. There are reports that 30 g a day or more can be used for acute illnesses. Burgerstein proposes a daily doses of 2 g, Linus Pauling up to 12 g for normal use. The body has one symptom that will show when the amount is sufficient: when the tolerance level has been reached diarrhoea occurs.

Drug addicts have an enormous deficiency — not only of vitamin C, but of vitamin and minerals in general. Consequently Burgerstein and the American authors propose giving multivitamins and multi-minerals as well as high doses of vitamin C. It is definitely worth taking the suggestions and experiences of ortho-molecular medicine into consideration when tackling such a complex and in-depth problem as addiction, but one should not fall into the trap of taking supplements instead of a healthy diet. A natural diet is the basic foundation of holistic therapy.

# VI. Bach Flower Remedies

Do not let yourself be prevented from using this method because of its simplicity. The further we progress in our research, the more clearly we will recognise the principle of simplicity in the entire creation.[62]

## Help for sick children

This therapy is unique and has proven its worth to such an extent that I would like to include it as an additional method of help.

Bach flower remedies have become increasingly popular in the past fifteen years, and are available in most chemists in Great Britain and continental Europe. His remedies are used worldwide by therapists, doctors and laymen and form part of many home first aid kits.

Dr Edward Bach (1886–1936), a successful English doctor, developed the Bach flower remedies after becoming an internationally renown researcher and homeopath. Even now seven nosodes discovered by him are part of the homeopathic repertoire, but he was never quite satisfied with what he had found, and searched for simpler solutions. He gave up fame, wealth and his surgery to move to the country and devoted himself to studying wild flowers. His wish was to substitute the intes-

tinal bacteria nosodes he discovered with plant remedies. He believed:

> The same as God in His greatness has given us food, he gave us beautiful flowers among the herbs of the fields that heal us when we are ill.[63]

Bach did not research the flowers according to their chemical properties and effects on the body, but rather according to their energetic characteristics that were able to influence positively our emotional state. His principle was simple and holistic: illness has more to do with our personality and emotional condition than with bacteria. It is our emotional and spiritual condition which governs our health. He believed that joy and enthusiasm are prerequisites for a healthy body. So he looked for plants to unlock our inner potential, liberate blocked life energy and convert damaging emotional attitudes.

Like homeopathic medicine, Bach remedies work on the level of 'information,' that is the energetic level. Each plant works through its specific characteristics on the individual's mood, and alters harmful behavioural patterns, which hinder development. As with homeopathy, no chemical substances are found in the water. However, Bach remedies are not made by succussion and potentization, but by infusing the plant in pure water and standing it in the sun at the place of collection or, in rare cases, by boiling the plant materials in water. Both methods are thus quite different from each other, and Bach remedies do not belong to homeopathic remedies, as many people believe. Classic homeopathy after Hahnemann, which is also concerned with spiritual and psychological symptoms, is extremely complex and needs a trained and experienced therapist. Bach flower remedies, on the other hand, were specifically devised to be used by lay people and for family use. Bach even stressed that he envied laymen who were able to recognize the underlying causes of illness without being hampered by medical knowledge.

There are thirty-eight different remedies plus the rescue remedy. As mentioned it is not the bodily symptoms which are treated, but the underlying mental condition which can hinder healing. This means that different people with the same physical problem need different remedies, as it is the cause which is being addressed. This could be, for example, lack of self-confidence, trust, feelings of guilt, homesickness, fear etc.

There are no known contra-indications for Bach remedies. It is not possible to overdose on them, and there are no side effects, even when taken over long periods of time. They can also be used in conjunction with chemical medicines. I have experienced exceptionally good results when using them for babies and small children. The children react well both with acute and chronic conditions. I often hear about midwives who have used Bach remedies during labour with good results for mother and child.

Since Bach remedies work on the emotional level they are an ideal measure for babies in intensive care or under observance. Bach remedies are also suitable as a supplementary therapy alongside conventional medicine. I cannot see any reason for not using them with children who are in hospital. We should be brave enough to discuss such wishes with doctors even though they may not by sympathetic. Many medical doctors do not believe in the dynamic forces of alternative therapies, but it is a shame to withhold help from sick children because of such attitudes.

## Flowers that can help infants

### Star of Bethlehem

Number 29 (*Ornithogalum umbellatum*)
I find this remedy one of the most important for infants. It helps with shock, for example birth trauma, separation, surgical procedures, hospitalization etc.

### Wild rose

Number 37 (*Rosa canina*)
The remedy for the condition 'inability to act'. It includes apathy, loss of joy for life, loss of energy, weakness, indifference, resignation after repeated disappointment.

### Honeysuckle

Number 16 (*Lonicera caprifolium*)
Remedy for homesickness.

Infants and children can be helped with this remedy if they suffer from homesickness or separation from their mother. Also if you have the impression that a newborn does not want to 'arrive here' properly.

### Aspen

Number 2 (Populus tremula)
Remedy for sudden fear, shaking, heart palpitations, withdrawal symptoms.

## Rock rose

Number 26 (*Helianthemum nummularium*)
Remedy for panic and fright. If the child is terrified: nightmares, surgical procedures.

## Olive

Number 23 (*Olea europea*)
Olive strengthens after a long illness, continuous difficult circumstances, after long-term strain.

## Crab apple

Number 10 (*Malus pumila*)
Helps to detoxify: after addictions, antibiotics and other drugs.

## Red chestnut

Number 25 (*Aesculus carnea*)
Remedy for a mother who worries continually about her child. Becomes more trusting and finds it easier to let go, for example when her child is hospitalized, when stopping breastfeeding, when the child goes to school etc.

## Rescue remedy

Rescue Remedy is kept in many home first aid kits and handbags. It is known for its instant effect. Mothers give it to their children for big and small injuries, trips to the dentist, for exams and general anxiety. Adults take it in stressful situations and for fear and challenges.

It can help a hospitalized child deal with fear, interventions, separation and shock.

> *Give Rescue Remedy to hospitalized infants and children before and after interventions and operations, for any kind of trauma, separation from their mother and fear.*

## Combinations of flower remedies

It is possible to combine different remedies. The following combinations are only four possibilities of many.

| | |
|---|---|
| 1. Star of Bethlehem Honeysuckle | For dealing with shock, homesickness and separation pain, strengthening |
| 2. Rock Rose Star of Bethlehem Crab Apple | For fear and panic, dealing with shock, de-toxifying after medication and addiction |
| 3. Wild Rose Star of Bethlehem | For giving energy and joy, resignation and loss of energy, dealing with shock |
| 4. Aspen Crab Apple Sweet Chestnut | Fear with shaking and/or sweating, detoxifying, after addiction, antibiotics, Desperation, loneliness, exhaustion |

## Preparing the remedies

If you do not have your own set of remedies you can buy single preparations in a chemist. They will mix you a diluted version of the remedy, or a combination of several remedies that you have chosen. Thus you do not need to buy the stock bottles.

If you own your own set, dilute as follows:
1 drop of concentrate of your chosen remedy to 10 ml of water, i.e. 3 drops to a 30 ml bottle.

The water used should be as pure as possible, for example, a good still mineral water or spring water if available. When diluting for adults and using tap water I add a few drops of cognac or vinegar to make the remedy last. The 'stock bottles' (the concentrate) can be kept for a practically unlimited amount of time. I find it better to use the dilutions within 3–4 weeks, and then prepare a new dilution. Dilutions seem to loose their effectiveness after some time.

## Dosage

> *4 Drops 4 times a day before or between*
> *meals and before bed.*
> *In acute cases 4 drops an hour*

The drops can be taken directly on the tongue or in a glass of water. Keep the drops in the mouth for a short time so that they can be absorbed through the mucous membranes. Infants are given their drops directly into their mouth with a pipette. Infants fed through a tube should receive 2 drops into their mouths.

Bach remedies can be given for as long as the condition persists, for a few days until the acute situation has passed, or for weeks or even months for lengthy problems. You cannot overdose.

The fact that it is not possible to overdose can lead to false assumptions. Do not underestimate the effect of the gentle flowers remedies. This method has proved itself worldwide for more than 50 years.

I hope this short introduction will lead to parents and doctors to take more note of these remedies, which can bring relief to babies. Once you know the remedies better you will not want to be without them. They are like a good friend who helps to overcome small and large obstacles. As these flower remedies work in a holistic fashion, they are not only useful in times of crisis, but also as a companion along the path of self-realization. They mirror aspects of our self that need to be transformed. They have the power to remove fears and attitudes that keep us from expressing our true, divine selves.

Bach remedy sets are available in many chemists. Those containing the 39 stock bottles are quite expensive, but can be used for a great many blends. I have treated hundreds of clients and used them for neighbours old and young — and my set is still not empty. Buying the set with several families or neighbours can make it more affordable and can also lead to an exchange of experiences and support with the different remedies.

# IV. Breaking the Cycle

## The inner path of the healer and educator

*Empathy, and the ability to love and share are not gifts of the intellect, but are the natural result of self-realization.*

We should remember that techniques are only guidelines and that treatments only develop healing powers by means of our involvement and empathy. If the methods bring joy and pleasure to you and your children, then you are on the right path. You will then find that your confidence increases, and that you can rely on your feelings more and more.

Treating and educating from a position of inner strength and maturity is more important today than ever. It is probably not an exaggeration to say that parents have never known and read so much about parenting and caring for children, and have never been able to give their children more. However, this does not seem to make it any easier. After an initial euphoric stage exhaustion often takes over, and daily family life is far removed from the ideal we carry in us.

Literature and further training do not auto-matically make us good parents. We all know from experience that neither knowledge from books nor a psychology degree guarantee happy relationships and families. It appears to be the same for parenting as for birth, of which Odent says we have never known so much and actualized so little. Everywhere we can see the same large discrepancy between what we know and what we are able effectively to achieve, and especially with children, where we try so hard but still get into difficulties or repeat the mistakes of our parents, which we strove diligently to avoid.

However, we are the children of our parents, and the past has shaped us. We carry the experiences and wounds of our childhood into our relationships, and they influence our behaviour whether we want them to or not. It is said that we pass on our wounds through seven generations! However, it is possible to break through this cycle. If we regard our problems as challenges — whether they are from family or work — they give us the chance to grow. We can learn more from our children than from anyone else; they force us towards self development. This seems to be the deeper meaning of every relationship and situation in life — they further our personal development.

What can help us to become good parents

and create the family we want for our children? We cannot obtain the quality of life we seek by giving in more often, acquiring more things or organizing more distractions and entertainment. We have tried that enough. We will not find the solution by granting our children more material wishes. Our children show us quite clearly that they are only more discontented.

The answer can be found on a different level and has to do with inner values. We are moved by a longing for real happiness and peace. Everyone wants to be happy. We are all surrounded by people who are longing for warmth, care, friendship and love. We need the companionship of other people. Even adults still have these basic needs. Part of us is, and remains, the small child that we were. And this inner child still has needs and desires. Western culture leaves little space for a child-like state, for spontaneity and playfulness. We have to be sensible and grown-up far too early. We suppress the desires, high spirits and adventurous nature of the inner child. However, yawning boredom cannot be relieved by television and computer games; they cannot fill the emptiness. We have lost the child-like curiosity and lively desire to find out about everything. We have parted from our joy of life and Godly wisdom that we had as a child. Erroneously, we see this as a sign of maturity. If one walks through the streets of a city most people appear unhappy and inhibited, but a reconnection with our valuable and spiritual child can make life exciting and rich again.

Overcoming old inhibitions and blocks will further our joy of life and release our inner riches. Our children need fulfilled, happy adults. The inner healing of parents and educators means more to our children than anything else we can give them.

I was allowed to make an important discovery in this regard and I hope that my experience might be of use to some readers.

I was the same as most other women, I knew I wanted children, was looking forward to having children and had plenty of time. But once I became a mother I found the task was not so simple. At first I was quite surprised, because I had looked after young cousins and neighbours from an early age. While working as an au pair in Britain when I was 19 I had been entrusted with the care of two sick babies, for whom I was responsible throughout the day. Thus I had gained lots of experience. However, I came across unexpected difficulties with my own children. I was more worried, and often plagued with feelings of guilt, which made me uncertain and inhibited me. I felt quite helpless.

At that point my subconscious helped me. One night, I had an remarkable dream, which changed the course of my life, and showed me many things about the connections in a mother-child relationship. In this dream I walked across a field, coming closer to a large swimming pool. I saw to my horror that my five-year-old daughter was lying at the bottom of the pool. It was difficult to say whether she was still alive or had drowned, because she was lying so still. I got such a shock that I woke up with a scream before I could jump in and save her.

At the time I could not understand what this dream was trying to tell me. I was puzzled why the drowning child was a girl. I myself did not have any daughters, but three sons. Then I was helped by a 'coincidence' — someone gave me a book about interpreting dreams.

I learnt from it that people and also objects in dreams are parts of our own personalities. Then the meaning of my dream became clear; I myself was the drowning girl! The dream was a clear message from my subconscious which I had to take note of: I needed to help the girl in the water who appeared to be lifeless. I also understood why. As a five-year-old child I experienced a dramatic escape from Germany with my parents and my family had been brutally ripped apart. The trauma had overshadowed my entire childhood.

After the dream I set out to help this inner child and to take its pain and wounds seriously. A daughter of C. G. Jung was my first helper in a process that took many years. She helped to clear my relationship with my mother, and I began to take over responsibility for my life without blaming anyone. After one session, which made important connections clear to me, I was able to understand my mother better and forgive her. After that something strange and impressive happened — two days after I had forgiven my mother I received a postcard from her. On the card a five-year-old girl was sitting beaming with her arms outstretched towards her mother, who was smiling and walking towards the child. My mother had sent the card the same day that I had experienced my inner breakthrough and had forgiven her! This is an example of how family members are connected and how a change in one person affects everyone else.

Several years later, after a lot of therapy and an exciting trip into my inner world, I was allowed to take my 'Godly' child by the hand in another dream. Or maybe the child was holding my hand?

Clearing our relationship with our mother and father is the most important thing we can do for the next generation. Things that have not been worked through influence our relationship with our own children. If we are able to experience gratitude towards our parents, and forgive them for our old disappointments and pain our relationship with our children will become deeper and more harmonious. Forgiveness seems to be the magic key. Through forgiveness we can remove obstacles which block our development and our ability to love. A definite sign that old wounds have healed, and that we have become free inside, is an increasing joy, which is unconnected to material goods and outer circumstances.

Good doctors, loving attentive parents and deep relationships do not stem from our intellect or from books. The ability to love is the fruit of self-awareness. Children need people who have *found* themselves. We should not underestimate the vast potential of a single soul. Once it has been realized, inner riches cannot be hidden. They shine like a strong light and illuminate everything in their path.

# Not enough time!

Only when I have become peaceful inside myself will I receive real knowledge. When I am calm primary power can flow through me, and I can listen to the voice of intuition. There is no better method of bringing harmony into my life than by arranging my daily deeds to bring me peace and calm.

I hope that the methods introduced in this book will help many children at home and those who need to be in hospital. Alternative medicines are well suited for use alongside conventional medicine in hospitals. The complementary partnership benefits everyone involved. The increased amount of time required is very worthwhile. One can be sure that much suffering — and also cost — can be prevented, in the health sector, in education and later in the fight against criminality.

However, we must practise what we know is good and necessary, and that is not an easy step. These things do not simply happen by themselves, and outer circumstances often stifle idealistic notions. All kinds of obstacles seem to appear. Lack of time — both in hospital and in home care — is often cited as the main problem. The feeling of never having enough time is part of life these days. The prevailing restlessness and business prevents much good. For some reason we seem to think that constant rushing and a full diary are signs of a fulfilled and efficient life. The more rushed and less available a person is, the higher their social standing seems to be, the more important their business. It would

be shocking to discover how much valuable, creative potential is lost because we are not able to access our talents and energy due to stress.

## Places of peace, sources of energy

Good care and good treatment need deep, individual attention. A doctor, nurse or therapist is personally involved in the process of healing. What we are able to give of our primal being to the meeting with another bestows the treatment method — whatever technique it may be — with the magical ability to heal. We should not become resigned or discouraged by lack of time, or other difficult external circumstances, or by the rigid structure of a work place. It sometimes appears as if, as a single human being, we have no effect on the problems with which we are confronted. In the economic sphere or workplace this may be true, but these are outer things. Our greatest strength comes from within, from our psychological potential. If we change our viewpoint from external circumstances to the laws of the inner world so-called *synchronicity* ensues — things flow into each other according to greater laws.

This means that we have the power to work from the inside against outer circumstances, and thus deepen our ability to heal. With a sensible, healthy and peaceful lifestyle we can strengthen these inner powers. If we strip ourselves of anything that robs us of our inner peace, and surround ourselves with people and things who bring us joy, we further our development. Creativity and wisdom derives from the peace at the centre of our being. From there the power to heal arises, as well as joyful calmness and confidence that our contribution is meaningful, and that we have the power to change things.

From the outside your life may appear to be humble and inconspicuous, but inwardly things will be moving. You will touch, inspire and encourage others through what you radiate. People will seek to be near you because they feel comfortable with you. Babies whom you have cared for during their illness will take more light with them through their life.

Carl Jung described this process in this way:

The great events in the world are basically of no consequence. Only the subjective life of the individual is of real importance. This alone makes history, in it alone all the great changes happen first, and all future and world history comes from the sum of all the hidden sources of individuals. In our most private and subjective life we are not only the sufferers, but also the creators, of a time. Our time — we are it.[64]

# Acknowledgments

I would like to thank the following people. They are part of the creation of this book, they have taught, inspired and accompanied me, and have given me practical help.

My thanks go especially to Dr Ruth Rice who taught me so much and whose research into the treatment of premature babies is so valuable.

My thanks also go to:
Marlis Holzmann, Pius Studer, Dr H. R. Suter-Blum, Peter Gmünder, Ellen Breindl, Georg Altermatt and Annegret Bohmert.

Teresa and her son Andrea for sharing her birthing photos and experiences with us.

Alin (and her parents) for letting us photograph her during massaging.

Chloe and her mother for their help with the polarity treatment.

Julia Woodfield, Scotland 2004

## Photographs

*Birthing photos*
Teresa Grütter and her son Andrea
*Baby massage*
Andy von Arx and Pius Studer

Illustrations on pages 87, 95, 96, 102, 103, and 105 by Lynne Denman, Wales.

# Endnotes

1  Dr Cicely Saunders, founder of the hospice movement

2  Chinese proverb

3  Horst Schetelig: *Geburt, Eintritt in eine neue Welt*, Verlag Dr Hogrefe, Göttingen

4  Ina May Gaskin: *Spiritual Midwifery*, Michael Odent: *Birth and Breastfeeding: Rediscovering the Needs of Women During Pregnancy and Childbirth*

5  Kennel et al: "Emotional Support During Labour," *Journal of the American Medical Assocation* Maxy, 1991

6  Liselotte Kuntner: *Die Gebärhaltung der Frau*, Marseille Verlag

7  Frederick Leboyer: *The Art of Breathing*

8  Adelle Davis: *Let's have Healthy Children*, Signet Books

9  Frederick Leboyer: *Birth Without Violence*

10  Jean Liedloff: *The Continuum Concept: In Search of Happiness Lost*

11  Swiss Radio DRS: Broadcast "Context", Baby-Power with Gisela Zeller-Steinbrich, broadcast on 15 July, 1991

12  Michel Odent: International Conference "Gebären in Sicherheit," Zurich 1992

13  Thomas Verny, John Kelly: *Secret Life of the Unborn Child*

14  Ashley Montagu *Körperkontakt* [*Touching: The Human Significance of the Skin*], p 68.

15  Ashley Montagu, p. 96

16  Ashley Montagu, p. 26.

17  Ashley Montagu, p. 26.

18  Frederick Leboyer: *Loving Hands: The Traditional Art of Baby Massage*.

19  Ashley Montagu

20  John Dobbing, *Developing Brain and Behaviour*.

21  Everett W. Bovard, *Effects of Early Handling on Viability of the Albino Rat*, Research Paper, 1958.

22  Michaela Glöcker & Wolfgang Goebel. *A Guide to Child Health*.

23  *Sunday Telegraph* (May 14, 1995) *Superbugs: Nature's Revenge*, Geoffrey Cannon.

24  Geoffrey Canon. *Superbug, Nature's Revenge*.

25  Amiel

26  Ruth D Rice. *Infant Stress and the Relationship to Violent Behaviour* (Lecture)

27  Lothar Burgerstein: *Heilwirkung von Nährstoffen* [Healing effect of food], published by Haug Verlag, p. 74.

28  Alex G. Schauss: *Orthomolecular Treatment of Criminal Offenders*, in Burgerstein, p.75

29  Herta Hafner. *Die heimliche Droge Nahrungsphosphat* [*The secret drug: phosphate in food*] D&M Verlag.

30  BBC news. 28 July, 1995.

31  Michael Odent: Lecture given at a conference entitled 'Gebären in Sicherheit,' Zurich 1992

32 M. Barth/U. Markus: *Zärtliche Eltern*, Pro Juventute Verlag.

33 Claire Gauch. *Die Macht der Zärtlichkeit* (*The Power of Gentleness*) AT Verlag.

34 Aletha J. Solter. *Tears and Tantrums: What to Do When Babies and Children Cry.*

35 Frederick Leboyer: *Birth Without Violence*

36 Carlyle

37 Frederick Leboyer: *Loving Hands: The Traditional Art of Baby Massage.*

38 Adelle Davis: *Let's have Healthy Children*

39 Susanne Fischer: *Medizin der Erde*, Hugendubel Verlag

40 Robert Tisserand. *Aromatherapy.*

41 Erik Sidenbladh: *Water Babies: A Book About Igor Tjarkovsky and His Method for Delivering and Training Children in Water.*

42 Judith Egli, Julis Emmenegger, counsellors for mothers: *Improving your own healing energies*. Self-published.

43 Video-Film: *The Kangaroo Care Method for Premature Babies,* The Amsterdam Civic Centre

44 'So warm wie im Kangurah-Beutel,' Article in *Krankenpflege* 8/93, S. Hamm, L. Stoffel

45 Susan M. Luddington-Hoe, Susan K. Golant. *Kangaroo Care: The Best You Can Do to Help Your Preterm Infant.*

46 Ruth Rice. "Effects of Rice Infant Sensorimotor Stimulation Treatment on the Development of High-Risk-Infants*,"* in G. Andreson and B. Raff (eds): *Newborn Behavioral Organization: Nursing Research Implications*, New York: Alan R. Liss, Inc. S. 7–26.

47 *Ibid*

48 Richard Gordon. *Quantum Touch: The Power to Heal.*

49 Video-Film: *The Kangaroo Care Method for Premature Babies,* The Amsterdam Civic Centre

50 Susan M. Luddington-Hoe, Susan K. Golant. *Kangaroo Care: The Best You Can Do to Help Your Preterm Infant.*

51 *Ibid*

52 ISPPM World Congress, Prenatal and Perinatal Psychology and Medicine, May 1992, Cracow, Poland

53 Ruth Rice: *The Kangaroo Method: Benefits of immediate and intensive Body contact of Mother with their Premature Infants,* ISPPM World Congress, May 1992, Cracow, Poland

54 Willy Brandt

55 Barbara Lukesch in *Weltwoche*, v. 18 June 1992

56 Soer und Stratenwerth, *Süchtig geboren, Kinder von Heroinabhängigen* S. 10, Rasch & Rohring Verlag. 1991.

57 J.L Halliday: *Psychological Medicine*, quoted in Montagu S. 65

58 Ashley Montagu: *Korperkontakt: Konzept der Humanwissenschaft*, Klett Verlag, S. 66

59 Dr Lothar Burgerstein. *Heilwirkung von Nährstoffen — Orthomolecular Medizin* [*Healing properties of nutritive substances — orthomolecular medicine*] Haug Verlag.

60 Bericht 1977. Libby & Stone: *The Hypoascorbemia-Kwashiorkor Approach to Drug Addiction Therapy*, in Burgerstein, S. 253

61 B Mäder: *Richtige Ernahrung*, glückerlicher Körper, Allsan Verlag, Seite 75

62 Dr Edward Bach. *Heal Thyself: An Explanation of the Real Cause and Cure of Disease.*

63 *Ibid*

64 C.G. Jung: *Mensch und Seele*, extracts from. Jolande Jacobi. Walter Verlag

# Bibliography

Bach, Edward. *Heal Thyself: An Explanation of the Real Cause and Cure of Disease.* C.W. Daniel Company, Ltd. Essex, 1998.

Burgerstein, Lothar. *Burgerstein's Micronutrients in the Prevention and Therapy of Disease.* Thieme Verlag. Stuttgart, 2002.

Cannon, Geoffrey. *Superbug: Nature's Revenge.* Virgin Books. London, 1995.

Chancellor, Phillip. *Illustrated Handbook of the Bach Flower Remedies.* C. W. Daniel Company, Ltd. Essex, 1996.

Davis, Adelle. *Let's have Healthy Children*, Signet Books. New York, 1981

Dobbing, John. *Developing Brain and Behaviour.* Academic Press. London, 1997.

Glöcker, Michaela & Goebel, Wolfgang. *A Guide to Child Health.* Floris Books. Edinburgh, 2003.

Gordon, Richard. *Quantum Touch: The Power to Heal.* North Atlantic Books. California, 2002.

Gaskin, Ina May. *Spiritual Midwifery*, Book Pub Co. Chicago, 2002

Jacobi, Jolande. *The Psychology of C.G. Jung.* Routledge & Kegan Paul. London, 1968.

Leboyer, Frederick. *Birth Without Violence* Element Books. London, 1995

— *Loving Hands: The Traditional Art of Baby Massage.* Newmarket Press. New York, 1997.

— *The Art of Breathing.* Element Books. London, 1991

Liedloff, Jean. *The Continuum Concept: In Search of Happiness Lost* (Classics in Human Development) Addison Wesley Publishing Company. Boston, 1986

Luddington-Hoe, Susan M. & Golant, Susan K. *Kangaroo Care: The Best You Can Do to Help Your Preterm Infant.* Bantam Books. New York, 1993.

Montagu, Ashley. *Touching: The Human Significance of the Skin.* Perennial. London, 1986.

Odent, Michael. *Birth and Breastfeeding: Rediscovering the Needs of Women During Pregnancy and Childbirth,* Clairview Books. London, 2004.

Sidenbladh, Erik. *Water Babies: A Book About Igor Tjarkovsky and His Method for Delivering and Training Children in Water.* St Martins Publishing. New York, 1983.

Solter, Aletha J. *Tears and Tantrums: What to Do When Babies and Children Cry.* Shining Star Press. Sussex, 2000.

Studer, Hans-Peter. *Vaccination: A Guide for Making Personal Choices.* Floris Books, Edinburgh 2004.

Tisserand, Robert. *Aromatherapy.* Harpercollins. New York, 1979.

Verny, Thomas & Kelly, John. *Secret Life of the Unborn Child,* Delta Trade Paperbacks. New York, 1982.

# Courses and Further Information

## United Kingdom

### Information on Baby Massage Courses for Parents and Carers

*Many hospitals and maternity units offer courses for parents and carers. Check with your local hospital for details.*

**International Association of Infant Massage (UK)**
72, Coningswath Road,
Carlton, Nottingham
NG4 3SJ
Tel/Fax: 0115 987 0655
Email: mail@iaim.org.uk
Web: www.iaim.org.uk

**Federation of Holistic Therapists**
3rd Floor, Eastleigh House
Upper Market Street
Eastleigh, Hampshire
SO50 9FD
Tel: 0870 420 20 22
Fax: 023 8048 8970
Email: info@fht.org.uk
Web: www.fht.org.uk

**Sure Start Unit**
Department for Education and Skills and Department for Work and Pensions
Level 2, Caxton House
Tothill Street, London
SW1H 9NA
Tel: 0870 0002288
Email: info.surestart@dfes.gsi.gov.uk
Web: www.surestart.gov.uk

### Professional Qualifications and Training

Chesterfield College, Infirmary Road,
Chesterfield, S41 7NG
Tel: 01246 500 562/563, Fax: 01246 500 587
Email: advice@chesterfield.ac.uk

Rochford Campus, Boston College
Skirbeck Road, Boston,
Lincolnshire, PE21 6JF
Tel: 01205 313218
Email: info@boston.ac.uk

Bishop Auckland College
Woodhouse Lane, Bishop Auckland
County Durham, DL14 6JZ
Tel: 01388 443000, Fax: 01388 609294
Web: www.bacoll.ac.uk

Blackburn College
Feilden Street, Blackburn, BB2 1LH
Tel: 01254 292149, Fax: 01254 292143

City College Birmingham
Soho Road, Handsworth,
Birmingham, B21 9DP
Tel: 0121 256 1102, Fax: 0121 743 9050
Web: www.citycol.ac.uk

City of Bath College
Avon Street, Bath, BA1 1UP
Tel: 01225 312191, Fax: 01225 444213
Email: hurstg@citybathcoll.ac.uk
Web: www.citybathcoll.ac.uk

East Riding College — Bridlington & Beverley
St Mary's Walk, Yorkshire, YO16 1JW
Tel: 01262 458800
Email: enquiries@eastridingcollege.ac.uk

Filton College
Filton Avenue, Filton,
Bristol, BS34 7AT
Tel: 01179 092319, Fax: 01179 312233
Email: sczeike@filton-college.ac.uk

Hartlepool College Of Further Education
Stockton Street, Hartlepool
TS24 7NT
Tel: 01429 295111, Fax: 01429 295000
Email: dcaygill@hartlepoolfe.ac.uk
Website: www.hartlepoolfe.ac.uk

Joseph Priestley College
Peel Street Centre, Peel Street
Morley, Leeds, LS27 8QE
Tel: 0113 307 6000, Fax: 0113 307 6001
Email: helpline@joseph-priestley.ac.uk
Web: www.joseph-priestley.ac.uk

Oxford and Cherwell College Of Further Education
Oxpens Road, Oxford
Oxfordshire, OX1 1SA
Tel: 01865 269269, Fax: 10869 248871
Email: enquiries@oxfordcollege.ac.uk
Web: www.oxfordcollege.ac.uk

Preston College
St Vincents Road, Fulwood
Preston, PR2 8UR
Tel: 01772 225484, Fax: 01772 25002
Email: dwatson@preston.ac.uk
Web: www.preston.ac.uk

Royal Forest Of Dean College
Five Acres Campus, Berry Hill
Coleford, Gloucestershire
GL16 7JT
Tel: 01594 838446, Fax: 01594 837497
Email: leslieb@rfdc.ac.uk
Web: www.rfdc.ac.uk

Saltash College
Church Road, Saltash
Cornwall, PL12 4AE
Tel: 01752 848147
Email: annette.luscombe@saltash.ac.uk
Web: www.saltash.ac.uk

Sandra Day School Of Health Studies
Ashley House, 185A Drake Street
Rochdale, OL11 1EF
Tel: 01706 750302, Fax: 01706 750304
Email: aroma@sandraday.com
Web: www.sandraday.com

South Lanarkshire College
Allers Campus
Kenilworth, Calderwood
East Kilbride, G74 3PQ
Tel: 01355 224801, Fax: 01355 228533
Web: www.south-lanarkshire-college.ac.uk

Stoke On Trent College
Cauldon Campus
Stoke Road, Shelton
Stoke On Trent, ST4 2DG
Tel: 01782 208208, Fax: 01782 603504
Email: gjone1sc@stokecoll.ac.uk
Web: www.stokecoll.ac.uk

Strode College
Church Road, Street
Somerset, BA16 OAB
Tel: 01458 844400, Fax: 01458 844411
Web: www.strode-college.ac.uk

The Holistic Training Centre
Abacus House, 1 Spring Crescent
Portswood, Southampton
Hampshire, SO17 2FZ
Tel: 02380 390982, Fax: 02380 390983
Email: markmcguinness@holistictrainingcentre.co.uk
Web: www.holistictrainingcentre.co.uk

# USA

## Information on Baby Massage Courses for Parents and Carers:

International Association of Infant Massage (USA)
1891 Goodyear Avenue, Suite 622
Ventura, CA 93003
Tel: 805 644 8524
Fax: 805 644 7699
Email.IAIM4US@aol.com
Web: www.iaim-us.com

## Training, courses and continuing education:

**International Institute of Infant Massage**
605 Bledsoe Rd NW
Albuquerque, NM 87107
Tel: (505) 341-9381
Fax: (505) 341-9386
Email: info@infantmassageinstitute.com
Web: www.infantmassageinstitute.com

**Associated Bodywork & Massage Professionals**
1271 Sugarbush Drive, Evergreen,
Colorado 80439-9766
Tel: 800-458-2267
Fax: 800-667-8260
Email: expectmore@abmp.com
Web: www.ambp.com
*To find a therapist in your area or a training program:*
**www.massagetherapy.com**

*Website with lots of information and advice on baby massage, including a "Holistic Premature Infant Massage Program" approved and recommended by Ruth Rice:*
**www.infantmassage.com**
Carla Steptoe
One-O-One
2822 Lawnwood Dr.
Ocean Springs, MS. 39564
Tel: 228-875-4140

## Other useful addresses:

**The Kangaroo Foundation**
Santafé de Bogotá, D.C. Colombia
Calle 56A No 40-02, Bloque A13, Apto 416, Pablo
VI edificios azules
Tel: 57 1 6083917
Fax: 57 1 2210731
Email: herchar5@colomsat.net.co
Web: http://kangaroo.javeriana.edu.co

*Contains a list of practitioners as well as details on schools that offer training in Polarity Therapy:*
**American Polarity Therapy Association (APTA)**
PO Box 19858
Boulder, CO 80308
Tel: (303) 545-2080
Fax: (303) 545-2161
Email: hq@polaritytherapy.org
Web: www.polaritytherapy.org

*Research into the benefits of baby massage:*
**Touch Research Institutes**
University of Miami School of Medicine
P.O. Box 016820
Miami Fl, 33101
(Located at Mailman Center for Child Development
1601 NW 12th Ave., 7th Floor, Suite 7037)
Tel: 305-243-6781
Fax: 305-243-6488
Email: tfield@med.miami.edu
Web: http://www.miami.edu/touch-research

# Index

# A Guide to Child Health

*Michaela Glöckler & Wolfgang Goebel*

This acclaimed guide to children's physical, psychological and spiritual development is now available in a brand new edition. Combining medical advice with issues of upbringing and education, this is a definitive guide for parents.

This book outlines the connection between education and healing, with all that this implies for the upbringing and good health of children. Medical, educational and religious questions often overlap, and in the search for the meaning of illness it is necessary to study the child as a whole — as body, soul and spirit.

The authors based their theory and practice on 17 years' experience in the children's out-patient department of the Herdecke Hospital in Germany, which is run along anthroposophical lines.

The first section covers childhood ailments and home-nursing. The second part looks at the healthy development of the child and how to create the best conditions for it. The authors go on to examine issues of upbringing and education, and their consequences for later life. Throughout, the book is extremely practical, with example situations of conflict and crisis presented, along with possible solutions. This new edition also includes medical and health practices in North America, Southern Africa, Australia and New Zealand.